Brief Therapy Conversations

W0113080

Brief Therapy Conversations features stimulating discussions between two international experts about essential topics, including the importance of the therapeutic relationship, the role of diagnosis, the therapist's mindset, specific techniques and guiding logics, therapist development, and likely future trends. It explores a wide range of literature and ideas on brief therapy and single-session therapy. For those interested in time-sensitive treatment, several expanded journal articles are included that provide additional insights into ways to improve therapeutic efficiency.

Reader friendly and conversational in format, this book is essential reading for professionals involved in brief therapy research, teaching, and practice.

Michael F. Hoyt, Ph.D., is a psychologist based in Mill Valley, California. He was one of the originators (with Moshe Talmon and Robert Rosenbaum) of the Single Session Therapy approach and is the recipient of various professional honors. He is the author/editor of numerous publications, including *Brief Therapy and Beyond*; *The Handbook of Constructive Therapies*; *Creative Therapy in Challenging Situations*; and *Single Session Thinking and Practice in Global, Cultural, and Familial Contexts*.

Flavio Cannistrà, Psy.D., is a psychologist based in Rome, Italy. He is the founder and co-director of the Italian Center for Single Session Therapy and of the ICNOS Institute, an international postgraduate training institute specializing in strategic and systemic brief psychotherapies. His publications include *Single-Session Therapy: Principles and Practices* (2021 in English, 2018 in Italian) and *Terapia Breve Centrata Sulla Soluzione: Principi e Pratiche* (*Solution Focused Brief Therapy: Principles and Practices*).

Brief therapy is best seen as a conversation. What better way, therefore, to unlock the mysteries of this way of working than through a series of conversations between a senior master and his most talented junior colleague? I cannot recommend this book highly enough. Both parts of the book are full of wisdom. If you buy only one book this year, buy this one.

Windy Dryden, PhD, is an emeritus professor of Psychotherapeutic Studies at Goldsmiths University, London, and the author of *Single-Session Therapy: Responses to Frequently Asked Questions.*

The conversations between Michael and Flavio elicit so much that makes therapy efficient and effective as well as compassionate and authentic. This book can help you to be a better therapist and maybe a better person.

Jeff Young, PhD, is the director of The Bouverie Centre and a professor of Family Therapy and Systemic Practice at La Trobe University, Melbourne, Australia, and the author of *No Bullshit Therapy: How to Engage People Who Don't Want to Work with You.*

This book is unique and full of wonderful ideas and suggestions. The authors cover an amazing number of subjects and ways of doing therapy, all of which are thoroughly documented in the footnotes and references. Readers will enjoy meeting the authors and listening in on their conversations.

Rubin Battino, MS, is the author of *Using Guided Imagery and Hypnosis in Brief Therapy and Palliative Care.*

This is a must-read for therapists and clients who wish to help and be helped effectively by psychotherapy. Michael F. Hoyt (representing the experienced elder of the tribe) and Flavio Cannistrà (representing the young and the eager to learn) have a great affinity and mutual respect for one another. Their conversations over the course of several years are inspiring, knowledgeable, and refreshingly clear and practical. They support the conversations with helpful guidelines and references to enrich greatly readers of all levels.

Moshe Talmon, PhD, is the author of *Single-Session Therapy: Maximizing the Effect of the First (and Often Only) Therapeutic Encounter* and *Single Session Solutions: A Guide to Practical, Effective, and Affordable Therapy.*

Brief Therapy Conversations

Exploring Efficient Intervention in Psychotherapy

Michael F. Hoyt and Flavio Cannistrà

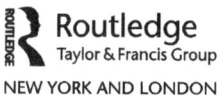
Routledge
Taylor & Francis Group

NEW YORK AND LONDON

Cover image: © Getty Images

First published 2023
by Routledge
605 Third Avenue, New York, NY 10158

and by Routledge
4 Park Square, Milton Park, Abingdon, Oxon, OX14 4RN

Routledge is an imprint of the Taylor & Francis Group, an informa business

Library of Congress Cataloging-in-Publication Data
Names: Hoyt, Michael F., author. | Cannistrà, Flavio, author.
Title: Brief therapy conversations : exploring efficient intervention in
psychotherapy / Michael F. Hoyt and Flavio Cannistrà.
Description: New York, NY : Routledge, 2023. | Includes
bibliographical references and index.
Identifiers: LCCN 2022015240 (print) | LCCN 2022015241 (ebook) |
ISBN 9781032310299 (hardback) | ISBN 9781032310282 (paperback) |
ISBN 9781003307709 (ebook)
Subjects: LCSH: Brief psychotherapy. | Psychotherapist and patient.
Classification: LCC RC480.55 .H6819 2023 (print) | LCC RC480.55 (ebook) |
DDC 616.89/147—dc23/eng/20220712
LC record available at https://lccn.loc.gov/2022015240
LC ebook record available at https://lccn.loc.gov/2022015241

ISBN: 9781032310299 (hbk)
ISBN: 9781032310282 (pbk)
ISBN: 9781003307709 (ebk)

DOI: 10.4324/9781003307709

Typeset in Garamond
by codeMantra

"To make progress toward doing therapy briefly, effectively, and over the widest possible range of problems, we must make a fresh start: in effect, to construct a new myth, a new view of problems and their resolution that is minimally constrained by past myths. On this view, both practice and thought basically should be exploratory."

—John Weakland (1990, p. 107. "Myths about Brief Therapy; Myths of Brief Therapy." In J.K. Zeig & S.G. Gilligan (Eds.), *Brief Therapy: Myths, Methods, and Metaphors*. Brunner/Mazel.) © Reproduced by permission of Taylor and Francis Group, LLC, a division of Informa plc.

To Jennifer and Flavia

Contents

List of Figures   ix
List of Table   xi
Acknowledgments   xiii
Preface   xv

PART I
Dialogues   I

1   The Therapeutic Relationship in Brief Therapy   3

2   Diagnosis and Brief Therapy   28

3   Mindset in Brief Therapy   52

4   Techniques and Logics in Brief Therapy   70

5   A Brief History of Brief Therapy, Some Personal Influences, and
     Thoughts about the Future   81

PART II
Extending the Conversation – Scholarly
Elaborations   121

6   Single Session Therapy: A Healthful Approach to Effectively
     and Efficiently Solving Client Problems   123

7 The 9 Logics Beneath Brief Therapy Interventions:
A Framework to Help Therapists Achieve Their Purpose 135

8 Common Errors in Single Session Therapy 157

Index 171

Figures

3.1   Context of Competence   67
5.1   Wall at MRI   84
5.2   Michael with Carl Whitaker, c. 1974   87
5.3   Michael with Bob Goulding, c. 1991   96
5.4   Michael with Steve de Shazer and Richard ("Dick")
      Fisch, c. 1994   103
5.5   Michael and Flavio with Botticelli's *Birth of Venus*   109
5.6   Skype screen shot, April 2020   112
6.1   Context of Competence   126

Table

6.1   Solution-Building Vocabulary   125

Acknowledgments

We express our deep appreciation:

- To our many teachers, colleagues, students, and clients for all they have taught us about effective and efficient intervention;
- To Sarah Gore and the editorial board at Routledge Publishers for embracing this project, to Georgina Clutterbuck for her attention to a myriad of editorial details, and to CodeMantra for their excellent production;
- To those who have permitted use of copyrighted materials;
- To Kaiser Permanente and to the APF Cummings Psyche Prize for support of Hoyt's studies and writing;
- To the Mill Valley Public Library for bibliographic assistance, to Darrell Coughlan for IT consultation, and to Roger Johnson and Phillip Ziegler for help with photos;
- To Federico Piccirilli, Angelica Giannetti, Pier Paolo D'Alia, Elisabeth Cinti, Valeria Campinoti, Beatrice Pavoni and Vanessa Pergher of the Italian Center for Single Session Therapy for creating with Flavio all the work around Single Session Therapy;
- To our families and friends for their love; and
- To one another for the pleasures of teamwork and good friendship.

  - Michael F. Hoyt, Mill Valley, California, USA
  - Flavio Cannistrà, Rome, Italy

Preface

In November 2015, then 34-year-old psychologist Flavio Cannistrà sent an e-mail from his office in Rome, Italy, to Michael Hoyt, a then 68-year-old American psychologist living in Mill Valley, California. Michael had authored and edited many books about brief therapy; Flavio, also a published brief therapy expert and the co-director of a postgraduate training institute, had various questions. Michael, still active as a teacher but recently retired from his many years of clinical practice, replied. A correspondence was begun.

A few months later, Flavio flew from Rome to the San Francisco Bay area to attend a two-day workshop Michael was teaching at the Mental Research Institute (MRI) in Palo Alto, CA. When Flavio walked in, they exchanged hearty *Ciao*s. After the workshop, Flavio stayed another day at the Hoyts' house in Mill Valley, and the two psychologists took a long day-into-night walk-and-talk. ("Similar, but not quite like when Freud first met Jung," they joked.)

Michael made two appearances, via Skype, in Flavio's training classes in Rome. Two books of his were translated into Italian (Hoyt, 2008/2018; Hoyt & Talmon, 2014/2018), and after nine months he traveled to Italy and co-taught a workshop in Rome for the Italian Center for Single-Session Therapy (with side visits to Naples, Pompeii and Firenze). Flavio's book *Terapia a Seduta Singola* (Cannistrà & Piccirilli, 2018) was published in Italian. A year later, another workshop, this time in Milan. Flavio then came back to the Bay area and was a speaker at a Brief Therapy Conference. They took a road-trip down the California coast from San Francisco through Monterrey, Big Sur, and Santa Barbara to Los Angeles. They coauthored a couple of articles for psychotherapy journals, and then they were speakers at the 3rd International Symposium on SST and Walk-In Services, held in October 2019 in Melbourne, Australia.

As readers of Jay Haley's (1985) three-volume *Conversations with Milton H. Erickson, M.D.*, Richard Simon's (1992) *One on One: Conversations with the Shapers of Family Therapy,* David Grove and Jay Haley's (1993) *Conversations on Therapy: Popular Problems and Uncommon Solutions*, or Hoyt's (2001) own *Interviews with Brief Therapy Experts* already know, friendly dialogue can be particularly useful for probing issues – questions can be asked, answers given, and responses can be revisited and reflected upon. At times, various parallel processes may emerge within the dialogues – process mirrors content, form follows function, and the medium becomes the message.

Brief Therapy Conversations: Exploring Efficient Intervention in Psychotherapy has two main parts. Some of the Hoyt-Cannistrà dialogues were recorded – on Skype, in the car driving along the California and Amalfi coasts, and also in Queenstown, New Zealand, after the 2019 Melbourne conference. *Part I: Dialogues* presents highlights from those conversations. Drawing on both American and European perspectives, five chapters offer practical information and in-depth reflections on topics including the therapeutic relationship; the role of mindset; the use of diagnosis and different techniques; the importance of culture; and perspectives on the history and future of brief therapy as well as discussion about mentoring and therapist development. It contains numerous clinical examples. Subsequently added footnotes, "gray box" highlights and chapter summaries enrich the discussion and provide further food for thought. *Part II: Continuing the Conversation – Scholarly Elaborations* carries on the discourse. It is comprised of three chapters, each an expanded version of a journal article by the coauthors – one about Single Session Therapy and some of its underlying principles; the second, about the logics that influence different efficient brief therapy interventions; and the third, a look at ways to increase or decrease efficiency, cast as a tongue-in-cheek list of ways to avoid success in single session therapy. Together, Parts I and II document a fertile collaboration and provide a rich array of learning opportunities.

Brief Therapy Conversations: Exploring Efficient Intervention in Psychotherapy is full of information and is a lively and fun read. It is intended as a professional book and also could be used in graduate school classes. With the current large and growing interest in brief therapy, both relative beginners and those more experienced who are interested in exploring ways to make therapy more effective and efficient will find much to consider. Readers will find an extended introduction to the principles and practices of brief therapy, how it works, and some of the most important authors. The themes discussed are of interest for every form of psychotherapy and will enhance understanding of where we want to go and how to get there.

References

Cannistrà, F., & Piccirilli, F. (2018). *Terapia a Seduta Singola: Principi e Pratiche*. Giunti (English version published in 2021 as *Single Session Therapy: Principles and Practices*).

Grove, D.R., & Haley, J. (1993). *Conversations on Therapy: Popular Problems and Uncommon Solutions*. Norton.

Haley, J. (1985). *Conversations with Milton H. Erickson, M.D.* (Vols. 1–3). Triangle Press.

Hoyt, M.F. (Ed.) (2001). *Interviews with Brief Therapy Experts*. Brunner-Routledge.

Hoyt, M.F. (2018). *Psicoterapie Brevi: Principi e Pratiche*. CISU (Centro d'Informazione e Stampa Universitaria di Colamartini Enzo) (published originally in English as *Brief Psychotherapies: Principles and Practices*. Zeig, Tucker & Theisen, 2009).

Hoyt, M.F., & Talmon, M. (Eds.) (2018). *Capturing the Moment: Terapia a Seduta Singola e Servizi Walk-In*. CISU (published originally in 2014 in English as *Capturing the Moment: Single Session Therapy and Walk-In Services*. Crown House Publishing, 2014).

Simon, R. (1992). *One on One: Conversations with the Shapers of Family Therapy*. Guilford Press.

Part I

Dialogues

Chapter 1

The Therapeutic Relationship in Brief Therapy

MICHAEL: I hear your voice and I can see you're looking at the screen. Let's make sure it's recording.

FLAVIO: I can see you and I can hear you. Can you see me?

MICHAEL: Oh yes! I can see you now – you're moving.

FLAVIO: Good – we're connected. Let's talk about the therapeutic relationship in brief therapy.

MICHAEL: Okay. I want to ask: How is Flavia? [Flavia is Flavio's girlfriend; she is a dance and Pilates instructor.]

FLAVIO: She's okay. She's working, she's starting a new course. She's fine.

MICHAEL: Good. I remember last time we were talking at the end of our meeting on Skype, she came walking in and she looked at me and she said: "Oh, Michael: your shoulders are different. A lot of exercise is helping."

FLAVIO: Yeah.

MICHAEL: So this got me to thinking about therapeutic relationships, because when I went the first time to visit my Pilates instructor we were talking and I was trying to decide: "Do I really want to get involved doing this with her? It's going to cost money, it's going to take time." We had a nice conversation, and then she said something that got me to say "Yes." I asked her about her training and her orientation and how long she was in practice and she gave good answers, and then I said: "How do you see the relationship when you are working with somebody?" And she said: "I am a movement wizard" – like a magician, a wizard – "My job is to use everything I know to see how to help you move better."

FLAVIO: Hmm.

MICHAEL: And right then I had the thought in my head, and it even came out of my mouth. I said out loud: "I am about to enter into a vulnerable relationship. I'm going to let my guard down and I have to let this person see me and how I'm not good at certain things." I'm trying now to figure out what was it that told me that it was okay. I think it was a combination. It was partly I wanted to find somebody to help me. So I was motivated. Partly she gave the right answers – she was smart, she was experienced. But then there was something about the way she said "movement wizard."

DOI: 10.4324/9781003307709-2

It made me feel that she's confident, she knows what she is doing. She is not going to just follow one approach. She's going to use different ideas. Her being confident gave me hope. She was not intimidated by me and my aching back.

FLAVIO: Once I was sitting in my office. I move a lot on my chair – up and down, here and there, I simply can't be in the same position all the time. That day I was moving maybe even more than usual, because a sun ray from the window was just blinding me! So I said to the client: "I'm sorry, I know, I always move a lot." And she said: "That's ok. That's you. You're authentic."

MICHAEL: Yeah.

FLAVIO: You know, and I think that having a good relationship is probably one of the most important factors in every profession. A friend of mine, a lawyer, when I asked her how to choose a good lawyer, she said: "One you trust. That's more important than how good he is." Relationship is trans-professional – regardless of the field, you need to have a good connection.

MICHAEL: Yeah. Both are important: You want them to be smart, but if you don't trust them you won't be able to work with them. So, I was thinking about the therapeutic relationship. Sometimes we meet somebody, and we connect with them … there's a rapport. Other times it seems stiff or we feel awkward or it doesn't feel like we want to "dance" with this person. So these are my thoughts about the therapeutic relationship, that there's a certain amount of trust that has to happen and there's something that happens between the two people that either encourages the alliance – you become allies – or it does not encourage it.

FLAVIO: Sometimes I hear people say "client" and sometimes they say "patient." In Italy, we also sometimes just say "person." How do you see the difference between "client" and "patient"?

MICHAEL: The terms *patient* and *client* are both used throughout the literature. It seems that psychoanalysts and psychiatrists and others working in medical settings generally prefer *patient*, which emphasizes the medical-model idea of expert-provided diagnosis and treatment, whereas others may favor *client*, to emphasize more egalitarian, collaborative/facilitative/strengths-oriented approaches. When I trained and worked in medical settings, I usually said "patient"; nowadays I usually say "client."[1]

I was thinking about lots of interviews and therapy sessions I've done with people and sometimes I'm serious and formal. Other times I'm laughing and I'm casual. I don't think it's just, "Do you smile?" There's something else. I'm not quite sure how to describe it, but there are certain people we want to be with them, they inspire us, we feel they have something to offer. What we talk about in brief therapy, our techniques, strategies, logics, all the different methods we use, we oftentimes assume that there's going to be a therapeutic relationship and it happens, but we don't really pay much attention to it. I think it's very, very important, particularly at the beginning, to form a good relationship.

Box 1. Therapeutic Relationship and Therapeutic Alliance

The relationship between a healthcare professional and a client/patient is the means by which a therapist and a client hope to engage with each other and effect beneficial change in the client/patient. The therapeutic relationship is considered in every approach to be one of the greatest contributors to therapeutic outcomes and one of its components, the therapeutic alliance, the most important predictor of therapeutic success. Relationship and alliance are especially influenced by the communication between client/patient and therapist.[2]

Some Alliance Building Questions

- How do you see or understand the situation?
- What do you think will help?
- How have you tried to solve the problem so far – how did that work?
- How can I be of help?
- If we were only going to meet once, what problem would you want to focus on solving at this point in time? (or: Given all the issues you've mentioned, which is the most important for us to focus on today?)
- Is this being helpful to you? What would make it more so?
- Are we working on what you want to work on?
- I might have missed something – what might that be?
- Do you have any questions you'd like to ask me?
- What needs to happen here today so that when you leave you can feel this visit was worthwhile?
- Do you know how to reach me if/when you want to be in contact?

There are lots of potentially useful alliance building questions, of course, and it is important *how* you ask the questions, as well – timing, warmth, humor, etc.

FLAVIO: So are you saying that in Brief Therapy we often take the therapeutic relationship for granted? It seems that way to me. I don't think we need complicated theories but maybe some more structured guidelines. You're one of the few brief therapists I've read who gives some structured guidelines about that.

MICHAEL: I like theory, but I think it's most important to be practical – otherwise, it may be philosophy but not therapy. I've gotten nice feedback that people have found the diagram showing the different phases of each session and the overall therapy, along with the list of questions[3] I developed to use at different junctures in therapy (pre-session, early, middle, late) to be very helpful – including questions to tune into the therapeutic alliance. We tend to focus on the relationship and alliance early in a therapy, but it is important to keep track of it throughout.

FLAVIO: The relationship is the base.

MICHAEL: Yeah. I've always liked the statement by Arnie Lazarus[4] that the therapeutic relationship is the soil in which techniques may take root.

FLAVIO: There's this research from Michael Lambert and from Barry Duncan and Scott Miller in which they talk about outcome variation in psychotherapy, and we know that thirty percent is explained by the therapeutic relationship. So it's important, of course, to talk about the therapeutic relationship, but sometimes it seems to me that we over-analyze it.

MICHAEL: Okay.

FLAVIO: The thing is that we capture some pieces (like "empathy" and "positive regard"), but we talk about them as if they are the only truth about therapeutic relationships. I read about John Weakland, about a "one-down" position,[5] and I thought: "Oh, that's good. This is a right way to do therapy. I do it and I make a good relationship with a client so probably it's true." *Probably*. It's true for *some* people, it's not true for *all* the people and it's true also for *some* therapists, but not for all the therapists, all the time. Sometimes we, as therapists, take some theories, some constructs, as absolutes that are always true or always useful – for everybody, for every situation. That is an epistemological error.[6] You know what I mean?

MICHAEL: If the client wants the therapist to be an expert authority, a classic professional, and if I tried to go one down, saying "Hey, call me Michael" and "Oh, I don't really know very much about this. Help me with this – what do you think?" they will not form a good relationship with me – they want an "Expert." But it can also be just the opposite, that if they want somebody who's more casual and friendly and if I act like a "Professional Expert" they will find me cold and distant. I think somebody like you or maybe somebody like me, somebody like John Weakland, we just know this. We don't have to think about it. We know how to get along with people. When we see somebody, we say: "Hi, how are you?" and by the way they respond, we know how formal to be, how close to stand to them, how loud, whether we should talk or mostly listen. It's very hard to explain it in words. It's like, how do we make conversation or how do you become a friend? How do you relate to people? And some people are much better at it, they just naturally get it – when you watch people, you see what they're doing.

So back to my Pilates – you'll see why I'm talking about this. I went out and bought a book called *The Complete Idiot's Guide to the Pilates Method*.[7] In the back, there was a section about the relationship between the Pilates instructor and the client. And they said it's very important to use the person's name a lot. "So, *Flavio*, we're talking about this, how are you today, *Flavio?*" And I noticed my instructor uses my name, so it becomes personal. It's about me. I also noticed that – just like you're doing right now looking at me on the screen – when I am doing some exercise, some pose or something, she's looking at me like I'm the only important thing in the world. Right then, she cares about me, nothing else. She's watching exactly what my arm does or my head does. She's paying a lot of attention and she uses a lot of positive reinforcement. She says: "Oh, that's good, Michael. There – you've got it." Even just the smallest little thing so that I feel like the more she sees, the better it is. So rather than feeling criticized, I feel welcomed and that she's accepting. And so I was thinking this is actually what we tell people to do in therapy: *Have positive regard, catch them doing something right, be supportive, don't be critical.*[8] Try to emphasize where the person wants to go, what are their best hopes, and help them to notice (and take) little steps along the way.

FLAVIO: Yeah, it's very crucial, as you say, to be connected with a person from the very first seconds — to look at her, to start to know her from the very beginning. I know that it's a matter of how you see the world, but sometimes for me it is simply astonishing, strange, reading about something like ten sessions, five sessions, to establish a good therapeutic relationship. I like when you say we can establish a good relationship in the first minutes, in the first five, ten minutes, by being interested, being curious, asking questions. It's strange because it seems to me that the main part of this big thing called "therapeutic relationship" is just that, you know what I mean? It's not everything, but the main part is "be with the person," with whom you have in front of you. But according to my university studies, a part of my mind still today says: "Is it really just this? Is it really just this apparently little thing?" I have a very good book, John Norcross' *Psychotherapy Relationships that Work*.[9] It's very interesting. It's very big. But it seems to me sometimes too much complicated for practice. I said that before: sometimes it seems to me that we're overanalyzing the therapeutic relationship.

MICHAEL: Like sticking a pin in a butterfly to study it better.

FLAVIO: Yes. It can result that when we're in front of the person we're not really there with her, we're following the book. And doing this, we also forget that there is not such a *thing* as the "therapeutic relationship." It's just a point of view. Useful, but just *a* point of view. Too often we forgot that we're working with constructs, that we invented the constructs and that we have to use the constructs and not be used by them. Do you know what I mean?

MICHAEL: Yeah. It gets complicated because if you're thinking much about "the seven dimensions," "the five characteristics," "the six techniques" – you're not present. You're not really there with the person. "Oh, tell me about yourself. What can I do for you?" To be intimate, you have to be "in-time-mate." Too much theory gets in the way of being immediate.[10] So, it's interesting to read a book, but I find sometimes when I have a checklist in my mind – "Are we doing this and is this unconditional positive regard?" – that it gets to be so much that I'm not talking to the person. I feel like I'm having a theoretical or philosophical exercise, but it's hard to reach people that way. "Hi. How are you doing? What's up?" Or maybe: "How can I help you?" or "Have I helped you?"

FLAVIO: Why do we complicate things so much? Because we're psychologists?

MICHAEL: Probably because we're psychologists and philosophers. Partly because Sigmund Freud wrote about transference and counter-transference: "What does it *really* mean and who am I *really*? What do I represent to them, their mother or their father? What's the *imago*? What's the unconscious image?" When things are going easy, what's different from the times when the relationship doesn't seem to flow or it's very difficult? That's why the guys in London[11] write that we should assume that the client is a *customer*[12] and our job is to figure out what they are a customer for, what they're looking for, rather than thinking they are a complainant or a visitor or resistant or don't want it. If the client is there they came for some reason and the idea is to find out, "How can I assist you or what would you like or what do you need from me?" And that's why I think solution-focused therapists like Harvey, Chris and Evan are so good at quickly getting involved and being helpful with people, because they say, "What's your best hope for today?" or "What would you like to get from today's meeting?"

FLAVIO: Solution-focused therapy is amazing. Their mission is amazing. I really can't believe that I could learn something so big, you know. If you ask someone if he is open-minded, probably he will say, "Yes" because nobody would say, "Oh, no I'm not." I was pretty sure about those things, but in my last trip in London I saw again things in a new light. First of all, I liked very much to consider every person as a customer.[13] If you have someone, if someone calls you and comes to you for therapy, if you don't have success in working with them, the problem is probably that you are trying to sell them your ways to see and to do things. You know what I mean?

MICHAEL: Yeah, in Zen Buddhism they say we are "selling water by the river." We're trying to give them themselves, but assisting them to look at themselves differently.

FLAVIO: Watzlawick said that people come to therapy and say, "Change me, change everything in my life, but just not *that* – and *that* is the problem I bring to you."[14] Probably sometimes when we do that it is because people come, and we want to change them in the way *we* think is good. This makes the resistance, you know? Sometimes, not every time. I think there is something else as well.

MICHAEL: *Resistance* means you are trying to get me to do something I don't want to do, so I resist. You try to control me or take over or make me do something I don't want. In psychodynamics the idea of resistance was that you were trying to get the patient to look at something they did not want to see, a feeling they didn't want to feel, a memory they didn't want to recall, so they would use "defenses" to resist or avoid going there if they didn't want to go to a certain place.[15] But "resistance" is feedback. We now treat resistance more generally as though resistance is just the person saying "No" and we have to find a way to join with them.[16]

FLAVIO: I like this definition, saying that the resistance is a reaction that a person has when you try to get her to where she doesn't want to go. Given the impossibility to reach a unique "deeper" explanation, it seems better if we stay on the surface of the problem, as de Shazer said,[17] working with it. At this point it becomes a matter of (a) *if* I have to bring the client to get there and (b) *how* to do that. This seems simpler and more useful to me.

MICHAEL: Yes. When we talk about the therapeutic alliance, alliance means we are allies, we are teammates, but we are allies with a common goal. What are we trying to accomplish together? How can I help you? What (and how) do you want to be different? What decided you to come to therapy? We have to remember there's a purpose and I think by bringing up the purpose and what they want different – "Oh, I can help you with that" – then the person becomes more open to talking with us because they see there's a reason to talk with us. They will get something from it.[18]

Let me ask something – I was thinking about this in a different way. You were just in London and you were at the BRIEF training and it was with mostly English people, British people. And you're an Italian. Do you have any ideas about how is it different to make an alliance in English with British people instead of in Italy with Italians? If I was going to come to Italy and try to do therapy and I said, "Flavio, what should I know to make a quick alliance with an Italian? Tell me what?" is there something I should say? Is there a certain way I should act? Do I look them in the eye? Do I shake hands? What's different between Italians and English? Of course, these are obviously big stereotypes.

FLAVIO: Very good question. Like Erickson said: "Observe, observe, observe." With English people, you need to give many more verbal feedbacks: "Oh, good. Yeah, that's fine." In Italy, in my experience, it's usual for me to be more moderate and to give fewer verbal feedbacks while the person is talking. And, another thing in England is to be more careful about the distance, you know, the physical distance but also the psychological, emotional distance, even a verbal distance. The sentence "Oh, this is very personal!" seems more common there in England than in Italy. I mean here (in Italy) it's not so common when considering a problem to ask for the person to disclose something "personal" – we just do that, that's all. It seems to me that the idea to be politically correct is more felt from British and Americans, too. In Italy you don't need to pay attention to every single word you say because of the racial or sexual implications. Sometimes it's really bad because there's a lack of awareness about how words work and also about important topics – for example, women's roles. Sometimes it could be good because there's a more relaxed climate. Italians tend to think that you said something in good faith and don't blame you. If you say, "Sorry, I didn't know," they will usually reply, "Don't worry. It's okay."

MICHAEL: OK. More active feedback with the English and more asking permission to talk about personal things. You have to be more: "Yeah, yeah. That's interesting."

FLAVIO: You know, in Italy we actually don't have many solution-focused therapists, neither books nor centers.[19] And many, many psychologists say that solution-focus doesn't work here in Italy because the culture is very different. Our culture is very different from English culture and the US culture, but now I can say that those psychologists were wrong. The culture is different, but solution-focused can work also in Italy. I'm more solution-focused than strategic, today. So, yes…

There's another thing that I connect to what we said before. I think that an approach like solution-focus is very difficult. I sometimes say that it's easy but not simple. It's easy because it's very easy to learn the fundamentals, but it's not simple because it's very complicated to do that very well. And an aspect is that you have really to listen to the person, to listen to what he or she wants. And this is so important also for the relationship. You simply can't say, "I'm the expert. You have to do this and that. This other is wrong and what I'm saying is right." Do you know what I mean? In other therapies, like strategic therapy, you do many things to *turn around* resistance. But now I can say you can do many things to turn around the resistance *you* created. And trying to turn around the resistance maybe you are making a bigger resistance. What I like in solution-focused is that if you assume that if something is good for the person, but if she says, "No, I don't like this. I don't want to do this. I can do that instead" then it's okay. "Perfect, we do something else."

MICHAEL: Yeah, it's not so simple. The idea is simple that we're going to look for the solution, but how do we do it? We are so trained to look for the problem instead of the solution, where you don't believe what they're saying: "What does it *really* say? What does it *really* mean?" It's like we're trying to find the code, we're trying to always interpret. There was the idea that somehow we have to diagnose, we have to find out what's wrong and we guide them from there. And the solution-focused therapists, they really let the client be the driver instead of the therapist.[20] But then, what do you do with these clients who say "Yes, but" and "No, but"? Who always, when you ask "Will you try this?" they say, "Oh, well, yes I could, but it won't work" or "No, I don't think that's a good idea" or "I did that once" or "I don't think I'm ready"? And the first time or the second time we think:

"Okay, I will go along." Then we begin to feel they just block everything. And then I was thinking, "So what are some of the things I have done in that situation?"

FLAVIO: Yes, I know what you mean. Sometimes *we* complicate things. We create a theory that helps us to explain certain things and to reach certain purposes. But then two things happen. First, we face the complexity of life, meaning that we face the truth that our theory is good to explain *certain* things and to reach *certain* purposes, but not the whole. And, second, we forgot we *created* a theory. We start to think that the theory is something that exists out there. So we complicate it. We create a more complex theory to explain other things and reach other purposes excluded by the first theory – and so on and on.

MICHAEL: Coming back to "Yes, but" people…sometimes it's a really good opportunity to go one down: "I've made different suggestions but I don't think I really understood. I was premature. Fill me in. What do you think would be helpful?" Of course, they may still reply, "Oh, I don't know – you're the doctor." In which case, "I don't know either. I suggested something, but I don't understand yet." So we can "Go slow," as John Weakland would say, or go one-down.[21] Sometimes it's a signal that the way we're working is not going to work. Maybe it's time to tell a joke.[22] For example, consider what effect hearing the following might have on someone who is not acknowledging his or her excessive drinking:

> A guy walks into a bar at 5 o'clock and says, "I'll have three beers." The bartender draws the beers and puts them in front of the guy and he drinks them, 1, 2, 3. The next day, the same thing – the guy comes in at 5, orders three beers and drinks them. After a few days of this, the bartender says, "You know, I could bring you the beers one at a time, so that each would be fresh and cold, rather than the three all at once" and the guy says, "Thanks, but the deal is this – every day when my two brothers and I are apart, at 5 o'clock we each go to a bar and order three beers and drink them – that way we can have a drink together every day." The bartender shrugs and says "OK." And for a while this happens: three beers every day at 5 p.m. Then, one day, the guy comes in and says, "I'll have TWO beers." And the bartender looks worried and hesitates – "Did something happen to one of your brothers?" And the guy says, "Oh, no – I've quit drinking!"

FLAVIO: *{laughs}*

MICHAEL: Or, it could be time to change the topic. We have to do something to better communicate, to change the energy and to change the mood. At MRI they were talking about therapist maneuverability, the therapist's maneuvers, one-up and one-down. "What would be best with this client?" And it's not always the same – even with one client. Sometimes we're one-up, sometimes we're one-down and sometimes we're level or symmetrical.

FLAVIO: What is the therapeutic relationship for you? How do you manage it during your work?

MICHAEL: Sometimes I will straight out ask people: "What kind of therapist would you like? One who listens, mostly? You want somebody who will give you advice? We could talk about things I think would make it better—but I think you already have some good ideas." What was helpful if they have been in therapy before? I'll say: "When you were in therapy before, what was helpful about that? What did the therapist do that you found useful?" Because they're telling me what works. You know, in solution-focused we say, "If it works, do more of it. If it didn't work, don't do it again. Do something different."[23] But if it works, do more of it. So I'll say, "Well, what kinds of things did you do with the therapist?" When they talk about what was helpful, they're giving me ideas of what kind of a therapist they want. I'm not sure I'm giving you a very good answer, though.

FLAVIO: I like the way you answered. Often, we will look for the theory of everything, the theory of all. Do you know this movie about Stephen Hawking, *The Theory of Everything*? I think that is the title in English. Stephen Hawking was looking for a theory that connected everything in the world. And he discovered that – at one point in his life he just said, "Yeah, it's impossible. There is not one theory for everything." So sometimes we look for something very, very simple, a simple explanation for everything. It's funny because before we were saying that sometimes, probably, the therapeutic relationship is something very simple. Now I'm saying that sometimes we are looking... for something that is too simple. I was thinking that while you were talking about the "Yes, but" people. Another thing is that sometimes we think, "You are the key." You just want to say to them something like, "Follow your path." But sometimes it's very hard because you find people that blame themselves or say, "I don't know. You're the doctor. Fix me." If I understood, in those occasions you try something to break the scheme, to shift the attention on to something else to stop what is going on in that moment. Is that what you do?

MICHAEL: If somebody counters by saying, "Well, you're the doctor," there are several options. Sometimes you could meta-communicate: "Let's look at what's going on between us. I make suggestions, but each time you tell me 'Yes, but' or 'No, but' – so I'm not sure what else I can offer you. How can I be of help?" So you talk about what's going on. Sometimes you can say to the person, "It may not make sense to you, but would you be willing to try just to see what happens? I don't want to explain it. I just want you to do it. Would you be willing to do that?" And it's an experiment. This happens with the Pilates teacher. She'll just move my arm this way or turn my body that way, and I could ask questions about anatomy – but usually I don't. I trust that she's giving me suggestions to do something for a reason. So sometimes we may say to our psychotherapy clients, "It would be better if you just try it, you'll see what happens." Sometimes that helps.

FLAVIO: Are there times or clients, I don't know, with whom you prefer to be direct? Because sometimes, it really helps to be direct to say, "Okay, probably you have to do that." Last week I saw two men. They are the brother and the husband of a woman who has a hoarding problem – you know, when you accumulate stuff, stuff, stuff ...

MICHAEL: OCD, keeping everything.

FLAVIO: Yeah, exactly. And they came and I really can say that they're very collaborative, but I really can't say why I felt that it was better to be very direct: "Okay, we have to do this and this and this and do that and do this, now." I didn't analyze why, but probably I was using feedback during the session. The question is: sometimes it's good to be direct, sometimes it isn't – right? Sometimes you need probably to be direct. I prefer the solution-focused way now, but I can see that sometimes you need something else. I liked it so much when Evan [Evan George, at the BRIEF training in London] said, "I try solution-focus for three sessions. If in three sessions I see no change I probably will try something else. I probably will start to think that solution-focus is not good for that person." This is very honest and very real. A pen is good for writing a lot of things but not everything. You can't paint Guernica with a pen. So, Single Session Therapy can be more directive than Solution-Focused: the model allows you to give suggestions, to suggest to her directly to do something, maybe because she recognizes you as a resource.

MICHAEL: If the person is in a *customer* (not *complainant* or *visitor*) position[24] and wanting information and professional guidance, why not? Some people want "professional guidance" and "expert advice." Of course, it's not going to work well to support *their* solution-building if you ask them what they think and then quickly switch to critiquing their thinking, or telling them what to do – in effect, you would be "Yes, butting" and "No, butting" them!

So the other day, I was talking with someone about anxiety. They called from New York City.

> I really would like to have one session with a therapist. I have anxiety. I have panic attacks, I get nervous before I do things, I start to sweat and perspire, I've been to therapy before and they want to talk about my childhood and all my relationships and I really just want some ideas and techniques of what could help me with my anxiety.

And I said, "Oh, when you don't have the anxiety, or when do you have it only a little bit, what do you do to control it?" So I started solution-focused: "What's the exception to the problem?"[25] And the person understood what I was doing, and she said, "If I tell myself, 'It's not so bad' or 'Don't scare myself, right, don't start to remember the worst thing that ever happened or the worst thing' I feel better." So here we were in a moment where in one way it's solution-focused therapy, but it's also about to be a cognitive-behavioral approach. I'm going to say, "Let me teach you how to think positive and how to use thought-stopping.

Let me teach you reframing and let me teach you breathing, relaxing muscles, different ways to reduce tension. We'll try different things and you can tell me which one of these works."

Some people would say, "You're being too direct, you're telling them" – but if it really helps, why not? If somebody comes and says, "I have trouble controlling my children. I need some parenting education" or "I have trouble sleeping. What can you tell me that will help me to sleep better?" I think they're asking us for information, and it's good to give them the information and see how they respond.

FLAVIO: We want the client to find his way, his solutions, his truth, his meaning. There are also important ethical implications. But sometimes, in some cases, it could be more effective to give a direction. What do you think?

MICHAEL: I do think you have to be careful because you want them, whenever possible, to think of the ideas themselves and make them their own. As the French philosopher Blaise Pascal said, "A thought is more likely to be accepted if it is perceived as arising in one's own mind." You don't want to undermine the client or foster unnecessary dependency. So it's not just "Tell them what to think." When I said to the person, "When you start to do something and get nervous, what is something you could tell yourself to stay calm?" she answered, "Well, I can remember the good time when it worked out okay." And so I "thickened" the story, asking for specific details: "Oh, good – what actually happened?" And she told me about a situation she was in and when she started to get nervous how she remembered to think positively. So, we try to help people get solutions as quickly as we can, and being directive may help them.

There are other patients that may say, "What should I do?" but they're going to respond with "Yes, but" or "No, but" to almost anything I say. There's a famous story about Milton Erickson, who was on one of his speaking tours, and he was going to demonstrate some sort of technique and he asked for a volunteer from the audience and a man raised his hand and started to come up – and Erickson recognized that this man was an opponent of Erickson.

Box 2. Milton H. Erickson, M.D. (1901–1980)

American psychiatrist who is legendary for his creative uses of communication and hypnosis to disrupt symptoms and evoke clients' resources to bring about therapeutic change. He is considered to be the "spiritual father" of various brief therapy approaches, including those developed at the Mental Research Institute, Neurolinguistic Programming, and Solution-Focused Brief Therapy.

*Quotable Quotes

1 "Each person is a unique individual. Hence, psychotherapy should be formulated to meet the uniqueness of the individual's needs, rather than tailoring the person to fit the Procrustean bed of a hypothetical theory of human behavior."[26]

2 "Patients have problems because their conscious programming has too severely limited their capacities. The solution is to help them break through the limitations of their conscious attitudes to free their unconscious potential for problem solving."[27]

3 "Emphasis should be placed more upon what the patient does in the present and will do in the future than upon a mere understanding of why some long-past event occurred."

4 "The patient comes to you with a certain mental set and they expect you to get into that set. If you surprise them, they let loose of their mental set and you can frame another mental set for them."

5 "And my voice goes everywhere with you, and changes into the voice of your parents, your teachers, your playmates and the voices of the wind and the rain."[28]

*Key Publications

M.H. Erickson (1980). *Collected Papers* (Vols. 1–4; E.L. Rossi, Ed.). Irvington.

M.H. Erickson, E.L. Rossi, & S.I. Rossi (1976). *Hypnotic Realities: The Induction of Clinical Hypnosis and Forms of Indirect Suggestion.* Irvington.

M.H. Erickson & E.L. Rossi (1979). *Hypnotherapy: An Exploratory Casebook.* Irvington.

M.H. Erickson & E.L. Rossi (1981). *Experiencing Hypnosis: Therapeutic Approaches to Altered States.* Irvington.

M.H. Erickson & E.L. Rossi (1989). *The February Man: Evolving Consciousness and Identity in Hypnotherapy.* Brunner/Mazel.

D.N. Short, "What is Ericksonian therapy: The use of core competencies to operationally define a nonstandardized approach to psychotherapy." *Clinical Psychology: Science and Practice,* 2021, 28(3), 282–292.

J.K. Zeig (Ed.) (1980). *A Teaching Seminar with Milton H. Erickson, M.D.* Brunner/Mazel.

J.K. Zeig (Ed.) (2021). *An Epic Life: Milton H. Erickson Professional Perspectives.* Milton H. Erickson Foundation Press.

He was very critical of Erickson. He didn't like Erickson's work. This is the story I've heard. And Erickson realized the man was coming up onto the stage not to cooperate, but to be difficult, to make Erickson look bad.

So, as the man walked onto the stage, Erickson said, "Since we have such a good volunteer, I am going to demonstrate how to work with resistance." And it's fantastic because the man is resistant. He's giving Erickson what Erickson wants, trying so badly to show no resistance.[29] Erickson has put him in a therapeutic double bind – the guy resists by not being resistant. Well, we have the same situation with some of our patients. If someone is being difficult or oppositional, I might say, "I'm wondering how you will say no to my suggestion. I'm wondering what are some of the ways you will find to not follow through. Will you not understand? Will you be too busy?" We have to be careful not to drive them off, but if they are resistant or they're opposing us, at least we make it obvious and difficult for them to continue doing it. Maybe we can capture them.[30]

FLAVIO: Yeah. I like this idea.

MICHAEL: Another famous Erickson story is the one about when he was a boy at the farm. I've heard there was a cow and he wanted it to go into the barn. And he was in front of the cow, pulling, trying to get the cow to go into the barn. But the cow was resisting, and Erickson couldn't get the cow to go in. He realized the cow was resisting – so what he did was he went behind the cow and he pulled on the tail. So then the cow walked forward to resist him – and walked right into the barn! So again, sometimes we have to outsmart the clients, trying to figure out how can we get them to resist in a way that will help them.

FLAVIO: Yeah. There is a thought that came up in my mind when you were saying something before. During my days in London, I gradually fell in love with solution-focused therapy. But there was a conflict because they said, "No, you don't give feedback to the person." With feedback I mean suggestions, advice, or something like that. I thought "But in Single Session Therapy we do that, it works. So, oh my God, what do I do now? Give or not give advice?" And I think that as you said a few minutes ago, it's just about doing what fits better with the person in front of you.

MICHAEL: If you give advice or do something other than work only with the client's own expertise, you may not be doing "pure" Solution-Focused Brief Therapy (SFBT) – but you may be getting the problem solved! At the end of his life, in his last great paper, "Analysis Terminable and Interminable," Freud[31] recommended alloying "the pure gold of analysis" with other base metals – meaning education, suggestion, advice, support, etc. – to make "a more durable therapeutic instrument." He spelled it out and acknowledged that it won't then be pure "insight"-oriented psychoanalysis – but also acknowledged that most people come wanting an efficient remedy and not "pure" psychoanalysis. Jay Haley had a case that he wrote about.[32] A mother brought her two children. The two boys were always fighting and difficult and Haley tried different things. He tried reinforcements. He tried punishment, he tried separating them. He tried all the usual things but nothing worked. Finally, he said, "If you don't do the bad behavior for one week, I will pay you $10." And he paid them and they stopped doing the behavior. People say, "How can you pay them?!" What it did was it disrupted the bad behavior and while they behaved okay for a week other things changed – like the way the mother responded to them. Change. The boys became friendly with one another. The whole context changed. So he didn't have to keep paying them $10 every week, but because this was an extreme situation, it was a way of saying we have to do something different otherwise it won't work – and this works. To my mind, the basic idea of solution-focused therapy is *do what works* and it's not unethical or criminal to sometimes give advice – or even sometimes medicine – if it is helpful and not harmful.

FLAVIO: It's very interesting because recently on Facebook a person criticized Single Session Therapy: "It's impossible to establish a relationship in one session. So it's impossible to help a person in one session." And I thought, "I have to call all my happy SST clients to tell them that they are not OK, they're still sick, their problem is still alive – even if *they* said that they're fine." What does a traditional therapist do during the first five sessions? What do they do to establish a relationship? I'd really like to be in their mind to understand what they see because it's another world, it's a very different way to see therapy and people and the relationship, you know?

MICHAEL: Some colleagues and I applied to give a presentation on Single Session Therapy at the American Psychological Association annual conference. We had given it other times before, and it had been well received. So we said, "We would like to give a symposium on Single Session Therapy." Three reviewers looked at our application. One was very positive. The second one was also positive. But the third one said, "Single Session Therapy cannot be therapy. It's speed interviewing, like speed dating, where you meet for five minutes." He actually said, "It's speed interviewing but it's not therapy." And they decided not to have us give the presentation. At first they just said "No." So I wrote back to the committee and I said, "Thank you. Could you tell us why not? So we can learn what to do differently next time. Or can you give us any feedback?" and then they gave us the feedback including the one person saying it was speed interviewing. So I wrote again and said, "Well, you know, there is a lot of evidence that one session helps many people, that it's not just speed interviewing" – but they already had their mind made up and I'm pretty sure they did not bother to look at the many studies or the different books I referenced. What this gets at is in the history of therapy, we developed the idea of working through, gradually forming an alliance, gradually working through the resistance, uncovering and going deeper, all of these ideas. And then somebody says "ONE session" or "brief therapy." If the theory of therapy is based on the idea that you have to gradually form an alliance and gradually uncover unconscious conflicts and gradually form a new relationship – and then something changes quickly, how do you explain that? That theory of therapy doesn't have a place for rapid change or quick change. And so I think the person, when he or she said it's speed interviewing, they were stuck in their framework and could not see the evidence because they already had made their mind up.[33] Sometimes we only can see what our theory allows us to see and there are theories that it must go slow and if it's quick then it can't be real. But it's interesting to have a lot of successful one-session therapy cases. And we usually don't spend much time interviewing the client about the therapy. What was most helpful? How did you know that we would be able to work well together? What did I do to make you comfortable? It will be interesting to get some of that information about when it worked quickly. How does the client understand how it worked?

FLAVIO: In this very moment we are doing a research very similar to your first research.[34] We sent a survey after every first session, a questionnaire online to the clients and we asked, "Did you ask for another session? Yes/No." And, "How much was the session helpful for you, from '1' (it wasn't helpful) to '5' (it was very helpful)?" And we asked, "How, why?" So we're asking an open question to understand why they found the session helpful or not helpful.

MICHAEL: James Prochaska has written about stages of readiness.[35] I think this is relevant here. Many people when they come for one session or for a brief therapy, they are ready to do something. They've been in the *precontemplation* or even *contemplation* stage, they are now *planning* their *action*, they're on the edge of doing something. And so we use whatever methods we use. We say, "Strike while the iron is hot," when it's ready. I think that's one of the reasons that brief therapy works: people come for brief therapy when they're ready. Maybe long-term therapy is really a lot of sessions getting the person ready for brief therapy!

So when I went to see the Pilates instructor, I had the thought I'm going to enter into a vulnerable relationship. That was the moment that the therapy began really, until then I was shopping and trying to decide, "Am I going to do this, or not?" And then I just felt confident this person could help me, I'm going to do it. I could have spent a lot of time interviewing other instructors or reading a lot of books, but instead something told me, "This is good, go for it." I think when people come for brief psychotherapy, oftentimes they come because they really want something. They're ready. "Why now did you come?" "I don't want it to continue any longer the way it is. I want to do something different." The Pilates instructor repeatedly said to me, "The more you do, the more you will get, the more you participate, the more you embrace this, the more practice you do, the more you will get out of it. We only meet once or twice a week in the office and you have the other five or six days and the other 23 hours."

I think the same thing is true in psychotherapy, encouraging them to participate: "How are you going to use this? Does that make sense? What are your next steps? Does that fit with what you came for? How does that go with your best hopes – does that fit the miracle picture?"

Flavio, I know you studied with Giorgio Nardone. So what does Nardone say about relationships and brief therapy?

FLAVIO: Yes, at the Centro di Terapia Strategica in Arezzo, Italy. In his first books, Nardone talks about the one-down position. But in a more recent book, now actually ten years ago, he said that it's important to have a therapeutic complementary relationship, you know, so you can have a one-down position or one-up position, and for some kinds of clients this is very helpful. He says that there are some relationships that work better for specific situations. For example, he says that with a phobic client, you know, with OCD, phobia, panic attack, an anxious person – he said that they often look for a technician, someone that in a very direct way says, "Do that, do this, do this thing, follow my path." With adolescents you need to be more ambiguous, back and forward, closeness and distance. With some kinds of anorexia you need to have a sort of "seductive" language – he means in a very ethical way, of course! You don't want to seduce your client – you just want to be perceived as fascinating.[36] He also says that there are four kinds of interactions. The first one is the collaborative one, people that follow you, everything you say. The second one is the "I would, but I can't." You meet them when you see people with panic attacks. "You're telling me to go out, to go around with people with my car, but I can't because I have panic attacks. So, you know, I would, but I can't." There's another one, the oppositional, people that would make a direct opposition: "I don't do this." Sometimes it seems like "I would, but I can't" but it's an opposition and with those kinds of client, Nardone says that you have to use a paradoxical relationship, like saying "Probably you can't do this" or "Probably I'm telling you something that you can't do"[37] or "I tell you: be more resistant, because it's very good for me," something like that. The last category is people that *can't* have collaborative relationships, like psychotics who can't be collaborative even if they want. This model is very useful. It taught me a lot. Like everything, it works for some things but doesn't work with everything. It's better to work with the assumption that the client is a customer and wants to work. If this mindset doesn't work, then you can start to consider his or her interaction, one of these four ways. I can try to use the "resistance" construct and then turn around the resistance with some kind of sophisticated linguistic technique. This is another example of how, to me, the constructs must be at your service and not you who must be at the service of the constructs.

MICHAEL: A patient who himself was a therapist came to see me. He said, "I understand you are going to fix me –" and then he laughed and said, "Let's see how good you are." I asked him, "What have you tried so far?" and he told me some things. And I said, "Well, if you've tried those, they are the ones I was going to suggest. So you have tried it already. If you were the therapist, and another person, a patient, came to see you, what would you tell them? Because you're the therapist." And he laughed and he said, "You're very clever. You're not going to let me trap you, are you?" And I looked at him and I said exactly this: "You're very clever and you're not going to let me trap you, either – so, now what should we do for the hour since we are going to sit here? And we're both very smart men who can make sure the other one doesn't do well." And he laughed and he said, "Well, you know, I really wanted to come and talk to you." He was having a problem with, I think, his girlfriend or somebody. And I kept saying, "What would a good therapist tell you?" By the end of the hour, he said, "This has really been helpful." He said, "I think what I see is that you got me to use my own ideas." And I said, "Well, I don't know if you're going to use them or not – that's up to you." And he laughed, and I said: "But you know, you still can pay for the session."

There are these difficult cases where sometimes people have had experiences – somebody who was an authority abused them, maybe molested them, at least was mean to them – so it's very hard for them to trust someone. And so sometimes I've found it helpful – and this is something many of my other brief therapy colleagues don't do – but sometimes I've made a psychodynamic transference interpretation.[38] I've said something like, "When I started to talk, you looked like you thought I was going to say something very bad." I might make a joke and say, "You looked the way I look when the dentist tells me they want to make a hole in my tooth." And they laugh and then I say, "Was that going on between us? From what you told me, it sounds like when other people have tried to help you or given you advice, it wound up hurting you. Do you think that's happening here?" And if they go, "No" I say, "Well, let's just watch and see if it happens." And then they become much more open-minded because they don't want to be seen resisting. I think it's really psychodynamic. I've made them aware of "You're saying 'No' to everything," so in a way it's meta-communicating. There are patients that I would just say, "I could explain this to you, but it would take a long time. But I think it would be better if you just tried doing this. It won't be perfect, but let's see what happens. Would you be willing to call your girlfriend and say this to her?" Would they be willing to read, you know, or do whatever the thing is I'm trying to get them to do? But these are the difficult patients, the "Yes, but" and the "No, but" folks.[39] I think there are other categories that are very good; they want to work with us. The ones who say "I would, but I can't," there are ways to work with that. "Well just try it and let's see how it goes wrong because we'll learn something." You can say, "I know you say you can't do it, but do it anyhow" – get them to act "as if."[40]

FLAVIO: What Nardone does with them is shift their attention: I give you a homework that seems to ask you something – but actually, I'm making you do something else that helps you to face the problems. For example, if you are a spider phobic, I ask you, "Okay. But how *much* are you phobic?" So next time you see a spider, you count the distance: "Tell me how much closer you can go to the spider. I just want to know the distance, so please don't go too close to the spider." This way works because I'm asking you to go toward the spider, to go close. I'm asking you to measure the distance, you know what I mean?"

MICHAEL: Getting them to begin to measure gets them to sit with and confront their anxiety, which is good. Sometimes we have to give them very specific directions. "I want you to look at that spider and just pretend that it is sitting there and then pretend it's a little bit closer." One of the things that Erickson would do, apparently, he would just assume that people were going to do what he said. Nowadays we are so politically correct and polite. We say to people, "Would you be willing to consider possibly trying maybe as an experiment…" We're inviting them but with all the qualifiers perhaps suggesting that they say "No." I would just say, "Imagine there is a spider sitting there." If you act as if it's just normal or okay to do it, sometimes people will follow us much more.

FLAVIO: This is a very important point, actually, because now we work in this time, and it's not anymore the age when the doctor was almost like God: "Whatever the doctor said, I have to do that."

MICHAEL: That reminds me of the joke about the pompous doctor: A fellow dies and goes to Heaven. St. Peter brings him in and is showing him around when the bell rings for lunch. Everyone gets in a long queue, but then one man just steps in front of the line and goes right in to eat. The fellow asks: "Who was that?" And St. Peter answers: "That was God – but he thinks he's a doctor!"

FLAVIO: [*laughs*] Right! Today it is not possible to have that kind of mindset and this is very important because we have to remember that we can't simply be fixed on doing what books say that were written 30, 40 years ago or 50, 100 years ago. In brief therapy, if we try to do the same things that Erickson did, even if in a personal way, we will have many problems. People have changed, things have changed and the world is changed.

MICHAEL: Some of the things they did, that Erickson did and then Haley did, nowadays people would say, "Are you crazy? No way, I'm not doing that. You can't tell me to do that!"

I had an interesting thought the other day. I'm writing chapters for a new book, and there was a case of mine that you may have read. There was a man [*goes into sonorous speaker's voice*]: "Sam was a 67-year-old man sitting in a wheelchair when I first met him at the HMO Clinic." That's how the case starts.

FLAVIO: Yes. It's in your book, *Brief Therapy and Beyond.*[41]

MICHAEL: Right. And then Sam comes in and he's had a stroke and he fears falling down and that he may not be able to get up and he's sitting in a wheelchair and we went into my office and we have a session. So when I was reading this, I had a "Oh my gosh, the case was 20 years ago!" realization. Twenty years ago! I said Sam was "67" or maybe I called him "elderly," and then I realized that now I am the same age that he was, actually a couple of years older – oh my gosh! And when I talked to him about his sons, and in the stuff we did in the office, he was an older man and I was a younger man. We had a bit of a father-son relationship. The reason I bring all this up is the alliance that we form with people depends on who we are at a certain time and now when people come to see me they see a grandfather or bald-head or an uncle or older gentleman or something like that, whereas 30 years ago or 20 years ago it was different. It made sense when I saw "Sam" for him to be the wise coach and for him to tell me how to do certain things, because that put him in the senior authority, expert adult role, compared to me. Part of what we did was I playfully threw myself on the floor and Sam repeatedly coached me on how to get up. If I did that with somebody now that would seem strange to them, it would not seem natural. "Why is this old man falling down on the floor in front of me and asking me how he should get up?" They would probably call 911 or the security guard! At the same time, 30 years ago, there were clients that I saw and they were older than me. I was half their age, so I did not have a lot of authority because I was younger. Now I meet somebody and because I look like the wise old bearded psychologist (ha!), I have a certain gravitas or charisma. You have to think of the therapeutic relationship. You can't just do what's in the book because the book doesn't say "He's sitting in a wheelchair" (or "You're sitting in a wheelchair"). People are going to respond to that person differently than to some young, strong, healthy-looking person. They're going to respond differently to a man than to a woman, to an attractive person versus a not-so-attractive person (whatever "attractive" means to them) and so on. So I think we have to figure out what kind of relationship can we form with people given who we are and who they are. It's individual for each. The general ideas are good: show interest, be kind, use their name, look for their strengths – they're good generalities. But when somebody says, "Well, how do you form a relationship with a bipolar patient? How do you form a relationship with a borderline? Or how do you form a relationship with a hoarder?" Well, how do you form a relationship with anybody? It's individual, it depends on who they are and who you are. So, Flavio – you teach, so you've had experiences. Somebody will raise their hand, and then they will say: "How do you get an alliance with a borderline who's been abused?" And you pause, then what might you reply?

FLAVIO: It would depend on who was asking, but maybe: "How do you do an alliance with a *person?*"

MICHAEL: *Va bene! Esatto!*

Box 3. Chapter I Summary: The Therapeutic Relationship in Brief Therapy

The therapeutic relationship and alliance are important factors in therapeutic change. The authors engage in dialogue exploring their implication in brief therapy. Emphasis is placed on the needs and ways to create collaboration and to deal with resistance. The importance of approaching each client individually is highlighted with clinical examples. Information is also provided about Milton Erickson.

Reflection Question: Describe something you did to form a productive relationship with a reluctant client.

Notes

1 See M.F. Hoyt (2017). "'Patient' or 'Client': What's in a Name?' and "'Shrink' or 'Expander': An Issue in Forming a Therapeutic Alliance." In *Brief Therapy and Beyond* (pp. 1–5 and pp. 217–218). Routledge. Carl Rogers (1951) popularized the term *client* when he named his famous book *Client-Centered Therapy* (Houghton-Mifflin). Nick Cummings (Cummings & O'Donohue, 2008, p. 91), however, pointed out the paradox that we may claim that "We treat 'clients,' not 'patients' [. . .] but [expect that] we should be paid by healthcare systems, both government and private, that are set up to take care of patients." N.A. Cummings & W.T. O'Donohue (2008). *Eleven Blunders That Cripple Psychotherapy in America.* Routledge. Also see M.F. Hoyt & S. Friedman (1998). "Dilemmas of Postmodern Practice Under Managed Care and Some Pragmatics for Increasing the Likelihood of Treatment Authorization." *Journal of Systemic Therapies, 17*(3), 23–33; reprinted in M.F. Hoyt (2000). *Some Stories Are Better Than Others.* Brunner/Mazel.
2 Bordin (1979) identified three components to the therapeutic alliance (sometimes called the *therapeutic relationship* or the *working alliance*): tasks, goals and bond. See E.S. Bordin (1979). "The Generalizability of the Psychoanalytic Concept of the Working Alliance." *Psychotherapy: Theory, Research & Practice, 16*(3), 252–260. Also see J.C. Norcross (Ed.) (2011). *Psychotherapy Relationships That Work: Therapist Contributions and Responsiveness to Patients* (2nd ed.). Oxford University Press.
3 See M.F. Hoyt (2017). "The Temporal Structure of Therapy: Key Questions Often Associated with Different Phases of Sessions and Treatments – Plus a Host of Helpful Hints." In *Brief Therapy and Beyond: Stories, Language, Love, Hope, and Time* (pp. 211–235). Routledge. For more on Feedback Informed Treatment (FIT), also see S.D. Miller, M.A. Hubble, & D. Chow (2020). *Better Results: Using Deliberate Practice to Improve Therapeutic Effectiveness.* APA Books.
4 A. Lazarus (1993). "Tailoring the Therapeutic Relationship, or Being an Authentic Chameleon." *Psychotherapy: Theory, Research, & Practice, 30*(3), 404–407.
5 See M.J. Lambert (1992). "Psychotherapy Outcome Research: Implications for Integrative and Eclectic Therapists." In J.C. Norcross & M.R. Goldfried (Eds.), *Handbook of Psychotherapy Integration* (pp. 94–129). Basic Books; and B.L. Duncan & S.D. Miller (2000). *The Heroic Client: Doing Client-Directed, Outcome-Oriented Therapy.*

Jossey-Bass. M.F. Hoyt (2019). "Going 'One-Down.'" In M.F. Hoyt & M. Bobele (Eds.), *Creative Therapy in Challenging Situations: Unusual Interventions to Help Clients* (pp. 103–112). Routledge.

6 See F. Cannistrà (2021). "The Vital Role of the Therapist's Mindset." In M.F. Hoyt, J. Young, & P. Rycroft (Eds.), *Single Session Thinking and Practice in Global, Cultural, and Familial Contexts: Expanding Applications* (pp. 77–88). Routledge.

7 K. Karter (2001). *The Complete Idiot's Guide to the Pilates Method.* Pearson Education.

8 As Goethe said in 1768, "Correction does much, but encouragement does more." Social psychologists Kenneth Ring and Harold Kelley (1963) documented the benefits of "augmentation vs. reduction training": rewards produce cooperation, and punishments and criticism produce concealment. As the old saying goes, "You can catch more flies with honey than you can with vinegar." Building on positives is usually more pleasant and reduces what is sometimes called "resistance." This is consistent with both Adlerian counseling and solution-focused brief therapy. See J.W. Goethe (1884). *Early and Miscellaneous Letters of J. W. Goethe: Including Letters to His Mother. With Notes and a Short Biography.* Reissued in 2009 by Cornell University Press; C. Flückiger & M.G. Holforth (2008). "Focusing the Therapist's Attention on the Patient's Strengths: A Preliminary Study to Foster a Mechanism of Change in Outpatient Psychotherapy." *Journal of Clinical Psychology*, 64(7), 876–890; K. Ring & H.H. Kelley (1963). "A Comparison of Augmentation and Reduction as Modes of Influence." *Journal of Abnormal and Social Psychology*, 66(2), 95–102; R.E. Watts & D. Pietrzak (2000). "Adlerian 'Encouragement' and the Therapeutic Process of Solution-Focused Brief Therapy." *Journal of Counseling and Development*, 78, 442–447.

9 J.C. Norcross (Ed.) (2011). *Op. cit.*

10 See C.A. Whitaker (1976). "The Hindrance of Theory in Clinical Work." In P.J. Guerin, Jr. (Ed.), *Family Therapy: Theory and Practice* (pp. 154–164). Gardner Press.

11 Flavio had attended a training with Harvey Ratner, Chris Iveson, and Evan George at BRIEF (formerly called the Brief Therapy Practice) in London. See H. Ratner, E. George, & C. Iveson (2012). *Solution Focused Brief Therapy: 100 Key Points & Techniques.* Routledge. Also M.F. Hoyt (2015). "Solution-Focused Couple Therapy." In A.S. Gurman, J.L. Lebow, & D.K. Snyder (Eds.), *Clinical Handbook of Couple Therapy* (pp. 300–332). Guilford Press.

12 See I.K. Berg (1989). "Of Visitors, Complainants and Customers." *Family Therapy Networker*, 13(1), 27.

13 Solution-focused brief therapy (SFBT) distinguishes *customers* (those wanting help and seeing themselves as empowered); *complainants*, those perhaps wanting help but not feeling empowered to make changes; and *visitors*, those who may be "visiting" but are not seeking help. See Berg (1989, *op. cit.*); also V. Shoham, M. Rohrbaugh, & J. Patterson (1995). "Problem- and Solution-Focused Couple Therapies: The MRI and Milwaukee Models." In N.S. Jacobson & A.S. Gurman (Eds.), *Clinical Handbook of Couple Therapy* (2nd ed., pp. 142–163). Guilford Press.

14 See "Constructing Therapeutic Realities: A Conversation with Paul Watzlawick." In M.F. Hoyt, *Interviews with Brief Therapy Experts* (pp. 144–157). Brunner-Routledge.

15 See A. Freud (1992). *The Ego and the Mechanism of Defence.* Routledge (Originally published in German in 1936; in English in 1966).

16 See S. de Shazer (1984). "The Death of Resistance." *Family Process*, 23, 79–93; also M.F. Hoyt & S.D. Miller, "Stage-Appropriate Change-Oriented Brief Therapy Strategies." In M.F. Hoyt (Ed.), *Some Stories Are Better Than Others* (pp. 207–235). Brunner/Mazel, 2000. For other discussions of the use of therapeutic contracts to minimize resistance, see E. Polster & M. Polster (1976). "Therapy without

Resistance." In A. Burton (Ed.), *What Makes Behavior Change Possible?* (pp. 259–277). Brunner/Mazel; and M.M. Goulding (1990). "Getting the Important Work Done Fast: Contract Plus Redecision." In J.K. Zeig & S.G. Gilligan (Eds.), *Brief Therapy: Myths, Methods, and Metaphors* (pp. 303–317). Brunner/Mazel.

17 de Shazer, S. (1994). *Words Were Originally Magic.* Norton.

18 See E. Polster & M. Polster (1976). "Therapy without Resistance." *Op. cit.* Also M.M. Gouding & R.L. Goulding (1979). *Changing Lives through Redecision Therapy.* Brunner/Mazel.

19 But now see F. Cannistrà & F. Piccirilli (Eds.) (2021). *Terapia Breve Centrata Sulla Soluzione: Principi e Pratiche.* EPC Editore. [*Solution Focused Brief Therapy: Principles and Practices*].

20 Added by Michael later: I recall in a conversation I had with Steve de Shazer and John Weakland (Hoyt, 1994/2001, p. 11) that Steve remarked that many therapists are "not 'mental health,' they're 'mental illness' professionals. It's not a mental health industry; it's a mental illness industry." I think Chris Iveson said it beautifully when he wrote (2019, p. 121):

> My professional world, the world of Solution-Focused Brief Therapy, is a topsy-turvy world where success still depends on trust – but on the therapist trusting the client rather than the other way around. Expertise is also crucial – however, it is the client's expertise, not the therapist's, that counts. Instead of the therapist understanding and solving problems, we have developed a conversational process which draws out and relies entirely on the client's knowledge to create new possibilities for their lives. Taking the radical position that we cannot know (or prescribe) the 'right' way forward for our clients, we have to trust their knowledge and treat them as the only experts in their own lives.

See M.F. Hoyt (2001). "On the Importance of Keeping It Simple and Taking the Patient Seriously: A Conversation with Steve de Shazer and John Weakland." In M.F. Hoyt (Ed.), *Interviews with Brief Therpy Experts* (pp. 1–33). Brunner-Routledge [work originally published 1994]. Also see C. Iveson (2019). "However Great the Question, It's the Answer That Makes a Difference." In M.F. Hoyt & M. Bobele (Eds.), *Creative Therapy in Challenging Situations: Unusual Interventions to Help Clients* (pp. 121–133). Routledge.

21 See M.F. Hoyt (2019). "Going 'One-Down.'" In M.F. Hoyt & M. Bobele (Eds.), *Creative Therapy in Challenging Situations: Unusual Interventions to Help Clients* (pp. 103–112). Routledge.

22 See M.F. Hoyt & S. Andreas (2015). "Humor in Brief Therapy." *Journal of Systemic Therapies*, *34*(1), 13–24.

23 From Hoyt (2001, p. 166):

> The basic rules of solution-focused therapy: (1)If it ain't broke, don't fix it. (2) Once you know what works, do more of it. (3)If it doesn't work, don't do it again; do something different. Following from these rules, some heuristic questions: *First session*—What do(es) the client(s) want? What can the client(s) do (toward what is wanted)? What needs to happen? *Later (second and subsequent) sessions* – What is better? What did the client(s) do (toward better)? What happened (to make it better)? What compliments and tasks can be given (staying within the client's expertise)? Is it 'better' enough – when should therapy stop?

See M.F. Hoyt (2001). "Solution Building and Language Games: A Conversation with Steve de Shazer (and Some After Words with Insoo Kim Berg." In M.F. Hoyt, *Interviews with Brief Therapy Experts* (pp. 158–183). Brunner-Routledge.

24 See I.K. Berg (1989). "Of Visitors, Complainants and Customers." *Family Therapy Networker, 13*(1), 27; and V. Shoham, M. Rohrbaugh, & J. Patterson (1995). "Problem- and Solution-Focused Couple Therapies: The MRI and Milwaukee Models." In N.S. Jacobson & A.S. Gurman (Eds.), *Clincal Handbook of Couple Therapy* (2nd ed., pp. 142–163). Guilford Press.

25 One of the basic tenets of SFBT is to do more of what works, and not do what doesn't work. What are the exceptions to the problem? Thus, a client may be asked to notice what is going on differently when the problem is not a problem, and to enact those differences. See M. Weiner-Davis, S. de Shazer, & W.J. Gingrich (1989). "Using Pretreatment Change to Construct a Therapeutic Solution: An Exploratory Study." *Journal of Marital and Family Therapy, 13*, 359–363.

26 J.K. Zeig (Ed.) (1980). *A Teaching Seminar with Milton H. Erickson, M.D.* Brunner/Mazel.

27 M.H. Erickson, E. Rossi, & S. Rossi (1976). *Hypnotic Realities.* Irvington.

28 S. Rosen (1982). *My Voice Will Go with You: The Teaching Tales of Milton H. Erickson.* Norton.

29 See M.H. Erickson & E.L. Rossi (1980). "Varieties of Double Bind." In E.L. Rossi (Ed.), *The Collected Papers of Milton H. Erickson* (Vol. 1, pp. 412–429). Irvington. Also see R. Bandler & J. Grinder (1975). *The Structure of Magic* (Vol. 1). Science & Behavior Books.

30 Michael adds later: I once had a patient who was very accommodating and had great difficulty asserting herself if she disagreed about something. I had recently taken a workshop with NLP developers Richard Bandler and John Grinder (1975) and had also read Erickson and Rossi's (1980) paper on therapeutic double-binds. When my patient denied we were disagreeing, I gently but firmly pointed out that right then we were disagreeing! She could then either agree that we were disagreeing, or disagree — either way, the linguistic structure resulted in realizing her difference from the therapist regardless of her answer. She acknowledged that we were having, as she put it, "maybe a difference of opinion" – and then added, "But that's a nice feeling to be able to say, 'I don't think so … it's not that way.' To me this is a big plus, down the street in the right direction." See M.F. Hoyt (1979). "Aspects of Termination in a Time-Limited Brief Psychotherapy." *Psychiatry, 42*, 208–219. Reprinted in M.F. Hoyt (1995). *Brief Therapy and Managed Care* (pp. 183–204). Jossey-Bass.

31 S. Freud (1937). "Analysis Terminable and Interminable." In *The Standard Edition of the Complete Psychological Works of Sigmund Freud* (J. Strachey, Ed.; Vol. 23). Hogarth Press, 1953–1957.

32 J. Haley & M. Richeport-Haley (2003). "Changing a Violent Family." In *The Art of Strategic Therapy* (pp. 79–95). New York: Brunner-Routledge. Cloé Madanes also reports a case in which a mother was paid to not hit her ten-year-old son. See C. Madanes (2006). "Money and the Family." In *The Therapist as Humanist, Social Activist, and Systemic Thinker … and Other Selected Papers* (pp. 97–117). Zeig, Tucker, & Theisen.

33 A controversy developed in 2019 in Ontario, Canada, when a regulatory board tried to deny Single Session Therapy (SST) hours as credits toward psychologist licensure. As Young and Jebreen (2020) detail, that wrongheaded effort was thoroughly debunked. See K. Young & J. Jebreen (2020). "Recognizing Single-Session Therapy as Psychotherapy." *Journal of Systemic Therapies, 38*(4), 31–44.

34 See F. Cannistrà, F. Piccirilli, G. Pietrabissa, P.P. D'Alia, A. Giannetti, L. Piva, F. Gobbato, R. Guzzardi, & A. Ghisoni (2020). "Examining the Clinical Incidence and Clients' Experiences of Single Session Therapy in Italy: A Feasibility Study." *Australian and New Zealand Journal of Family Therapy, 41*(3), 271–282.

35 J.O. Prochaska (1999). "How Do People Change and How Can We Change to Help Many More People?" In M.A. Hubble, B.L. Duncan, & S.D. Miller (Eds.), *The Heart and Soul of Change: What Works in Therapy* (pp. 227–255). APA Books.

36 Nardone et al. (2018, p. 62) talk about a "Seductive shake-up of emotions and reinforcement of the patient's confidence in her own beauty":

> While it is true that a male therapist might induce an emotional stirring, a female therapist can be a seductive behavioral model that the young woman can imitate. Consider, for example, the considerable 'seductive' qualities of therapists such as Virginia Satir, Mara Selvini Palazzoli, and Cloé Madanes, to name just a few.
>
> G. Nardone, R. Milanese, & T. Verbitz (2018). *Prisoners of Food: Research and Treatment of Eating Disorders*. Routledge.

37 Also see R. Fisch, J.H. Weakland and L. Segal (1982). *The Tactics of Change: Doing Therapy Briefly*. Jossey-Bass.

38 One size (or method) doesn't fit all. Better to be *multitheoretical*, asking "What would be most useful with this client and this therapist in this situation at this time?" Techniques can be eclectic but should be used toward a purpose – as we discuss in Chapter 4 and at length with many examples in Chapter 7.

39 Rubin Battino (in Hoyt & Battino, 2022) reports another method for dealing with people who repeatedly say "Yes, but…" or "No, but…":

> One of my favorite approaches […] is to tell the client that I am at my wit's end in helping him, and that the only way out of this impasse is to switch roles. So, we change seats and act each other. It is important to use the client's language, posture, emotions, and manner of speaking. It is even more important to overdo and exaggerate their behavior since this is actually a mini 'psychodrama' of their life.

Battino goes on to give a case example:

> At that point I said 'Harry, let's switch roles. You be me, and I'll be you.' I proceeded to complain and complain and 'Yes but' and 'No but' until Harry laughed and said 'Stop! I get it.' When I responded, 'No – I'm the client. I don't care if it's screwing up my life – I'm going to do it more and more and you can't stop me,' he replied: 'Okay, I'm being impossible – I'll stop being a jerk.' And he did desist from his counterproductive ways.

See M.F. Hoyt & R. Battino (2022). "On the Importance of (Occasionally) Being Unpredictable." *The Milton H. Erickson Foundation Newsletter, 22*(1), 12.

40 "As if" is a therapy technique, originally developed by Alfred Alder and now used in a variety of approaches, in which the client is encouraged to act as though the problem is solved (e.g., they are no longer afraid) or as though ("as if") they already have a quality (e.g., "courage" or "social popularity") they wish to embrace. Enacting the behavior provides them with the experience and also leads others to see them and respond to them in the desired way. "Fake it until you make it" thus can become intrapsychically and interpersonally self-fulfilling. See R.E. Watts, P.R. Peluso, & T.L. Lewis (2005). "Expanding the Acting As If Technique: An Adlerian/Constructive Integration." *Journal of Individual Psychology, 61*, 380–387.

41 On pp. 62–65 in M.F. Hoyt (2017). *Brief Therapy and Beyond*. Routledge. A report of the same case also appears on pp. 107–109 in M.F. Hoyt & M. Bobele (Eds.) (2019). *Creative Therapy in Challenging Situations: Unusual Interventions to Help Clients*. Routledge.

Chapter 2

Diagnosis and Brief Therapy

FLAVIO: Okay, we're recording.

MICHAEL: You said that you would like to talk about diagnosis and brief therapy, right?

FLAVIO: Yes.

MICHAEL: Why?

FLAVIO: Why?

MICHAEL: I think it's an important subject, but do you have a particular question?

FLAVIO: It's something that I face very often with my colleagues. Brief therapy is seen as something revolutionary, it's very different from many traditional things that we call "therapy." And a big difference has to do with diagnosis. Brief therapy is more interested in the process of change, and if we do an "assessment," it is different from many dominant therapies. Did we do well by avoiding traditional diagnosis? We should probably review the concept of *diagnosis*, and question ourselves deeply about differences in its use within the medical model and within psychotherapy. This discourse is often not touched in brief therapy books. When I studied at university, my textbooks and my professors said, "You need to do diagnosis, because without a diagnosis you can't do therapy." And colleagues interested in what I do, they say, "What about diagnosis?" And often I don't do a diagnosis in that traditional sense. I don't do the full assessment, the tests. I don't use the scales and so on. So, my first question – there are a lot of questions opening in my mind – the first question is, "Where is diagnosis in brief therapy textbooks?" I've read many brief therapy books – you've probably read many, many more books than me – but it seems to me that there is not much about diagnosis in brief therapy books. So, in brief, I would like to know if you, with your experience, have the same opinion, and if so, why?

MICHAEL: I have several ideas about it. Let me start at the top.

FLAVIO: Okay.

MICHAEL: The word *diagnosis* comes from the Greek words "dia" and "gnossis." "Dia" means "passing through" or "way" (like "via") and "gnossis" means

DOI: 10.4324/9781003307709-3

"knowledge." So a useful "diagnosis" should give us a way or information that would help us help the client.[1] A lot of diagnosis seems to me very discouraging. Saying that the patient is "borderline," "depressed," "obsessed," is calling them names, but it doesn't really help us figure out what to do to help the client and it doesn't talk about the client's strengths.

FLAVIO: That reminds me also that the past president of the DSM-IV Task Force, Allen Frances, said something like that diagnoses are everything but objective.[2] And Michael White was just one of the many therapists who warned us of the risk of using those labels.

MICHAEL: Here I want, as we say in English, to talk out of both sides of my mouth. Giving a pejorative label is counterproductive, but I think diagnosis sometimes can be helpful. I like to know things about clients, but I think a lot of diagnosis comes from us trying to be like medical doctors, thinking that we should be able to make a diagnosis so that we know what medicine to give them. What dose? How many treatments? How many sessions? Steve de Shazer did not like the idea of diagnosis at all.[3] When I asked him a question like "What about a borderline patient?" he said, "I don't know what that means, 'a borderline patient.' I don't know what that means. What is the problem? What is the exception? What would be helpful for them?" Milton Erickson also famously said, "I wish that Rogerian therapists, Gestalt therapists, transactional group analysts, and all the others would recognize the therapy for person #1 is not psychotherapy for person #2."[4] So even when you get a diagnosis, you then still have to figure out now what am I going to do?

Just because they have (or qualify for) the diagnosis of "OCD" or "schizophrenia" doesn't tell you really what to do. Some approaches have tried to develop protocols: "Here's what you do for OCD, here's what you do for depression, here's what you do for a particular sexual problem," whatever. Then you need a diagnosis because you look it up in the book, and the book tells you "This is the treatment." Many years ago I had a teacher who said to me, "You'd better diagnose the patient quickly before you get to know too much about them!" He meant that once you get to know them, they will become a person and you will no longer see them simplistically as "histrionic" or "depressed," so you need to do it quickly.

FLAVIO: A diagnosis can actually be a "complexity reducer,"[5] it can take you quickly to beaten paths. And surely we all feel calmer – professionals, institutions and perhaps even clients – in knowing that we are giving a name to something, a name that will allow us to follow the paths that, in the past, have led to results. But perhaps at this point the problem becomes: "But *which* diagnosis? That of the *DSM*?" Because there are different ways of doing diagnosis. Different *dia-*, different *ways* that lead you to different *-gnosis*, to different kinds of knowledge.

MICHAEL: Karl Tomm, the family therapist, wrote a paper[6] in which he said that the *DSM*, the diagnostic and statistical manual, is "spiritual psychosis."

He said, and I agree, it robs the person of their humanity. You're putting them in a category rather than working with that person. Someone else[7] wrote a book called *I Am More than My Label* about working with severe mental illness. "I'm not just schizophrenic, or whatever – I am more than my label." Irvin Yalom,[8] who is a psychiatrist, acknowledged that diagnosis is critical in treating severe psychiatric conditions with biochemical substrates but also pointed out that "diagnosis is often *counterproductive* in the everyday psychotherapy of less severely impaired patients." There is an interesting book by Jeffrey Lieberman about the history of psychiatry's attempts at diagnosis – he says that diagnosis involves a complicated brew of theoretical obligations, professional guild issues, monetary interests, and efforts at medical science.[9] In the United States, if you want insurance to pay for the treatment, you usually have to have a *DSM* diagnosis. Long ago the American writer Ambrose Bierce wrote this very funny book[10] called *The Devil's Dictionary* in which he gave this cynical definition: "*Diagnosis.* noun. A physician's forecast of disease by the patient's pulse and purse."

FLAVIO: This is interesting! A *DSM* diagnosis. It's good to remember that the *DSM* is a product of a specific professional association. It reflects its point of view and its interests.

MICHAEL: Definitely. Oftentimes they'll say that otherwise it's not a "real condition requiring treatment," it's just a "problem in living." So sometimes you have to get a diagnosis. When I asked Steve de Shazer,[11] he said if you need to have a diagnosis, have someone else interview them for the diagnosis and then come in and talk about therapy; or put on a white coat, like a doctor, and say "Now we're going to do the assessment" and then take off the white coat and say, "Now we're going to figure out how to help you." He separated diagnosis from therapy.

Box 4. Steve de Shazer (1940–2005)

Principal developer (with Insoo Kim Berg and others) of Solution-Focused Brief Therapy (SFBT). He was a constructive minimalist who modeled how effective therapy works rather than proposing a theory of mental illness. His approach is based principally on asking questions to help clients find their solutions to problems and to create different perspectives about their situation.

*Quotable Quotes

1 "Where you stand determines what you see and what you do not see; it determines also the angle you see it from; a change in where you stand changes everything."

2 "Problem talk creates problems, solution talk creates solutions."

3 "The miracle question was not designed to create or prompt miracles. All the miracle question is designed to do is to allow clients to describe what it is they want out of therapy without having to concern themselves with the problem and the traditional assumption that the solution is somehow connected with understanding and eliminating the problem."

4 "The three rules of SFBT: (1) If it ain't broke, don't fix it. (2) Once you know what works, do more of it. (3) If it doesn't work, don't do it again; do something different."

SFBT Questions

- *The Skeleton Key Question* (to elicit information about pre-session change or improvement): "Between now and the next time we meet, I would like you to observe, so that you can describe to me, what happens in your _____ that you want to continue to have happen."

- *The Miracle Question* (to enchant and orient toward the positive and to identify the goal of treatment): "Suppose that one night, while you were asleep, there was a miracle and this problem was solved. How would you know? What would be different?"

- *Exception Questions* (to identify times the presenting problem has not been present): "When in the past might the problem have happened but didn't (or was less intense or more manageable)?"

- *Endurance (or Coping) Questions* (to acknowledge difficulties and pains while still focusing on strengths and competencies): "Given all that you've been through, how have you managed to keep going as well as you have?"

- *Agency (Efficacy) Questions* (to identify clients' abilities to make a difference in the desired direction): "How did you do that?" or "How did you get that to happen?"

- *Scaling Questions* (to measure clients' own perceptions, to motivate and encourage and to elucidate goals and progress):

  > "On a scale of 1 to 10, 1 being absolutely no [*pick one:* hope, motivation, progress, etc.] and 10 being complete [hope, motivation, etc.], what number would you give your current level? What will tell you that your level has gone up one level?"

*Key Publications

I. K. Berg (1994). *Family-Based Services: A Solution-Focused Approach*. Norton.

I. K. Berg & Y. M. Dolan (2001). *Tales of Solutions: A Collection of Hope-Inspiring Stories.* Norton.

S. de Shazer (1982). *Patterns of Brief Family Therapy.* Guilford Press.

S. de Shazer (1985). *Keys to Solution in Brief Therapy.* Norton.

S. de Shazer (1988). *Clues: Investigating Solutions in Brief Therapy.* Norton.

S. de Shazer (1991). *Putting Difference to Work.* Norton.

S. de Shazer (1994). *Words Were Originally Magic.* Norton.

FLAVIO: I think this is right. The first thing that came to my mind is that when we talk about diagnosis, often we are talking about nosographical categories. With the *DSM*, you look at categories of symptoms and you find the symptoms and then say: "Okay, you have this label." As I said before, this is *one* kind of diagnosis. There are also, for example, psychodynamic diagnoses. In systemic or strategic therapy they talk about *operative diagnosis*[12] – they are more based on interaction and they observe how a person reacts, believing that you cannot really know a complex reality if you have not understood how it can be changed.[13] But when you think about diagnosis and when you study at university, you mostly study the nosographic diagnoses. And you learn to think that is THE diagnosis, but it's an error. But in the present that is the most common kind of diagnosis, and in society we use this diagnosis for bureaucratic things, for example, as you said, to go to an insurance company for money.[14] So that's a piece of reality and you can use it for something but, as you said, you have to have in mind the question if these kinds of diagnoses allow us to do our best therapy.

MICHAEL: If we use the term *diagnosis* more generally to mean a way of assessing what is needed (or "knowledge that points the way") I think then "diagnosis" can be helpful and, in fact, sometimes necessary and inevitable. Years ago I was having a public conversation about constructivism with Scott Miller, Barbara Held and Bill Matthews at an Erickson Brief Therapy conference.[15] And Barbara made the cogent point that it is very hard to have a method of therapy that doesn't have implicit within it some idea of what the problem is. She pointed out that even if your idea is to help the client deconstruct their text to give them a new narrative, there is the general implication that you think the problem is how they are linguistically constructing their experience – and you proceed accordingly. I think so. How and where you look influences what you see and what you do. As you said earlier, Milton Erickson counseled, "Observe, observe, observe." If you think, à la MRI (Mental Research Institute), that the problem is unsuccessful attempted solutions that actually serve to perpetuate the problem, you give directives to interdict and disrupt those attempted solutions; if you think, à la SFBT, that the problem is the client is persisting in something that doesn't work, you try to get them to "do something different." We may theorize globally, but we act locally. I recall having a conversation with Paul Watzlawick,[16] in which he said that he had found it very useful to totally abandon diagnostic terms; instead, he suggested, one should learn to speak the client's language (their way of looking at things) and to recognize that every system is its own best explanation. de Shazer thought of his approach more as a model that guides therapist and client pragmatically toward *what works* rather than as a theory of therapy based on the diagnosis of some putative underlying pathology.[17]

FLAVIO: I've read *The Great Debate in Psychotherapy* by Wampold and Imel.[18] I agree with them that a common result of all the psychotherapies is a change of meanings, so we need information about those meanings. Sometimes it is better to act on the client's meanings first to change their behavior, other times it may be better to act on their behavior first to change her meanings later. So we use this information to (1) understand the patient's meanings (to speak his/her language); and (2) to use those meanings to produce a change (in the "meaning to behavior" way or in the "behavior to meaning" way).

MICHAEL: When we select an intervention from the list of "9 Logics"[19] we're not doing so randomly — we have formed some sort of idea that this is what is needed. So when somebody asks, "What is the diagnosis?" I'm thinking, "What system of diagnosis do you mean? How will that help me with therapy?" When you're making a global *DSM* diagnosis — like *borderline, narcissist, obsessed* — how is that going to help me know what to do? In some systems of therapy, there are these protocols, what you should do; but then others say, we don't even need to know because our approach is "non-normative"[20] and each person is an individual. We're trying to enter their reality and looking for their strengths, their abilities.

FLAVIO: I think this is a huge shift in perspective, yet I'm not sure that professionals and institutions are ready to receive it. "We have always done so" is one of the most common forms of resistance — and the reality is that it does not come from clients but from us.

MICHAEL: Should therapists only work with certain kinds of patients? "I'm an expert on OCD. I'm an expert on schizophrenia." Or, can we work with a wider variety because we're looking for the client's strengths and resources? Even inside of diagnoses, there are secret strengths. For example, the person we say is *obsessive*, we could also say is very good at noticing small details. The person who is *dependent* is very good at taking instruction. The person who is *histrionic* is very emotionally sensitive. The person who is *paranoid* is very good at identifying who can help them and who might hurt them. So, when I hear a diagnosis it's good to consider "What is good about having that diagnosis?" It's not just "What is bad about it?" I would not say, "Oh, you're a narcissist" to the person, but if you're a narcissist you're someone who is very proud and will want to do a very, very good job in therapy. If you're depressed, you like to go slow and think about things deeply and you don't want to be rushed. So is there a way, if you're going to diagnose the person, to see and use the secret strength and to see what's positive in the diagnosis rather than just seeing it as a problem?

If I do a full assessment, I have to ask them about their childhood and their parents, their thoughts, their sleep, their sex life, their appetite, their traumas, their disappointments, their failed jobs, their moods, their relationship problems. It can be very depressing for the client and very depressing for the therapist.

FLAVIO: Here is another interesting point. Traditionally, we make diagnoses as we do in medicine, looking for signs and symptoms, but we do not ask, "What impact does this investigation have on the person?" Well, what impact does the psychological or psychiatric diagnosis have on the patient?

MICHAEL: Right. If "How you look influences what you see," looking for everything that's wrong is really going to discourage the person: "You thought you had Q, but you also have X, Y, and Z." IF (big "IF") you're going to use the *DSM* I think it's good to share it with your client: "I was thinking this diagnosis might fit – in the last six months, have you had 6 of the following 9 symptoms," etc. We can talk about a label in a way that doesn't encourage the person to over-identify with it.

Almost nobody comes to therapy because they have "schizophrenia." They come because "something is bothering me" or "I don't have friends." Almost nobody comes because "I have narcissism." They come because "I'm lonely" or "Nobody respects me." I think it's important to recognize that people who have schizophrenia also have life: "Oh, I can't get a date," or "I keep hearing a voice telling me that I should hurt somebody" or that "I'm dirty." They have a specific problem that they want help with. So I think it's always important to ask, "What is the problem that brought you here? What will tell you things are getting better? What would tell you we don't need to keep meeting because the problem is no longer a problem?" Otherwise we're trying to cure "borderline-ism" or "narcissism."

FLAVIO: Suddenly the diagnosis disappears and we are there with the person, finally. But at this point I wonder: what happens to the shortcuts? If I no longer have a diagnosis, how do I know which previous attempts to address that problem have proved useful so I can follow them? Actually, I would like to say that the diagnosis does not disappear, what disappears is the nosographic diagnosis as the *only* way to understand the client's problem. We could have another system that tells us how to work with certain dysfunctional behaviors and with certain strengths. It would become another diagnostic system, perhaps more useful but to be tested.[21] I wonder if there will ever be interest in this. The point, however, seems to me to be that we should help the person, not to treat a diagnosis.

MICHAEL: Exactly. I remember I was at a conference one time and I heard somebody ask Jay Haley, "Oh, I have a borderline patient who has attention deficit disorder and depression and..." They gave a long list, and Jay said: "I would not let that be the problem. A problem is something that has a solution. So why are they there and what do they want help with?" His point was, they don't want help with "borderline." They want help with "I get too upset" or "Nobody likes me" and what to do.

Box 5. Jay Haley (1923–2007)

One of the "first generation" major developers of family therapy, systemic-strategic interactional therapy, and brief therapy. He was a coauthor of the famous "double-bind" paper (Bateson, Jackson, Haley, & Weakland, 1956[22]); the founding editor of the journal *Family Process*; the person who most brought Milton Erickson to wider recognition; and the author of numerous foundational brief therapy texts. He created Strategic Family Therapy, a problem-solving approach focused on reorganizing family hierarchies in a more functional way.

*Quotable Quotes

1 "Therapy can be called strategic if the clinician initiates what happens during therapy and designs a particular approach for each problem. When a therapist and a person with a problem encounter each other, the action that takes place is determined by both of them, but in strategic therapy the initiative is largely taken by the therapist. He must identify solvable problems, set goals, design interventions to achieve those goals, examine the responses he receives to correct his approach, and ultimately examine the outcome of his therapy to see if it has been effective. The therapist must be acutely sensitive and responsive to the patient and his social field, but how he proceeds must be determined by himself."

2 "If therapy is to end properly, it must begin properly – by negotiating a solvable problem and discovering the social situation that makes the problem necessary."

3 "This is not a therapy where relationships are changed by talking about relationships but by requiring new behavior to solve a problem. [...] Giving directives, or tasks, to individuals and families has several purposes. First, the main goal of therapy is to get people to behave differently and so to have different subjective experiences. Directives are a way of making those changes happen."

4. "We once assumed that long term therapy was the base from which all therapy was to be judged. Now it appears that therapy of a single interview could become the standard for estimating how long and how successful therapy should be." [23]

*Key Publications

J. Haley (1963). *Strategies of Psychotherapy*. Grune & Stratton.

J. Haley (1969. *The Power Tactics of Jesus Christ and Other Essays*. Avon Books.

J. Haley (1973). *Uncommon Therapy: The Psychiatric Techniques of Milton H. Erickson, M.D.* Norton.

J. Haley (1977). *Problem-Solving Therapy: New Strategies for Effective Family Therapy*. Jossey-Bass.

J. Haley (1984). *Ordeal Therapy: Unusual Ways to Change Behavior.* Jossey-Bass.

J. Haley (1985). *Conversations with Milton H. Erickson, M.D.* (Vols. 1–3). Triangle Press.

J. Haley & M. Richeport-Haley (2003). *The Art of Strategic Therapy.* Routledge.

M. Richeport-Haley & J. Carlson (Eds.) (2010). *Jay Haley Revisited.* Routledge.

FLAVIO: This can be very disturbing for a psychologist because they traditionally teach us in a different way. They teach that there are sicknesses, there are ills and we have to treat the illness. There are many implications. For example, you can't have a single-session therapy[24] because illness implies that you need many sessions, that you can't treat that problem in one session. So here is another element that appears from our speech: a nosographic diagnosis implies a label that also contains rules about itself. If you are "borderline" you will require years and years.[25]

MICHAEL: Another problem is that, following from the medical model, a diagnosis can eliminate the person of the therapist.

FLAVIO: What do you mean?

MICHAEL: There is often the implication that there is a standard psychological treatment to apply once the patient has been diagnosed. Like once you do the right medical test and have the medical diagnosis (e.g., what kind of bacterial infection), there is a "right" medicine (e.g., penicillin) and any doctor can prescribe it. In psychotherapy, the "common factors" research evidence[26] says that it is the client and the relationship (people!) that are most important, not the technique. Psychotherapy is a creative human process. It can be studied scientifically, but it is conducted (we can hope!) personally and artistically.[27]

Sometimes we talk about personality disorders. A "personality disorder" means the person has a way of thinking, feeling and relating that significantly and repeatedly interferes with social, occupational, and family functioning. Sometimes one session may help but if they keep having the same problem over and over they may need more than one session to help them see the world differently and to learn to relate differently. Like in that case[28] you described so well in the book I coedited with Monte Bobele – it took time for the client to really learn to see things differently and to respond differently. So, I think we have to be careful that we don't try to say to people we can solve every problem in one visit. But we also have to deal with what the client, the patient[29] wants to deal with rather than, "Well, you think you have this problem, but you really have this much bigger problem. And we have to meet forever and ever and ever."

FLAVIO: Maybe we can shift the focus and see what is the specific reason the person came now. As Jeff Young[30] has written, Single Session Therapy (SST) is a service delivery system. So, I don't want to treat the so-called personality disorder. "I want to help you with the things you tell me you need to be helped with. So my door is always open. You can come back every time you want from one, ten, a hundred sessions."

MICHAEL: I think that's much better than to tell the person at the beginning, "You need a hundred sessions."

FLAVIO: A friend of mine is a CBT therapist and psychologist and he loves tests and he's very, very good. He often does the MMPI, the Beck Depression Inventory, these kinds of instruments. He told me a few days ago, "What about the prognosis?" He said: "I did some personality tests with the client and from those tests, I predicted that he probably will have had this kind of behavior" and he's right. Of course, you are not a magician, but we can predict something. What do you feel about this aspect of diagnosis?

MICHAEL: I once wrote a big paper about diagnosis,[31] and then over time I began more and more to realize that most people come for one session or three sessions and we have to help them with their problems right now, and that personality disorder diagnosis is so global that it doesn't help a whole lot.

FLAVIO: This reminds me of when Jeff Young pointed out to a public health service that in their four initial assessment sessions they lost 40% of the patients, thus suggesting they start with the SST and *then* do the four assessment sessions if necessary.

MICHAEL: If you ask the right questions and listen, the client will tell you what they want. In a discussion we had with John Weakland, Steve de Shazer[32] once said, most therapists are mental-illness professionals, not mental-health professionals. We don't look at their health, we don't try to bring out the best. We mostly try to get rid of the problems. So that influenced me as I began to do more very brief therapy. But I also see what your colleague was saying, that if we see that the person is likely to have certain problems, it's good to know that, just like I might, while addressing the problem they specify, treat someone somewhat differently if that person has obsessive compulsive disorder.

We can get stuck in the problem of *either/or*: either we diagnose them or we don't, either it's good or it's bad. Back to the beginning: what kind of diagnosis will help us help the person? Will it show us a way we can help them, or does it just condemn the person by using professional language to say that they're really badly damaged?

FLAVIO: Yes. It is in these situations that I say we have a "pragmatic approach." Not simply "do this" because the guidelines, the university, the theory you have decided to belong to – this is a beautiful phrase: "I belong to a theory," whereas the theory should belong to us and be at our disposal –

MICHAEL: – Lynn Hoffman talked about the "lenses" through which we look, and Mark Hubble and Bill O'Hanlon talked about "theory countertransference."[33]

FLAVIO: It tells me to "do so," but because what you are doing is giving you results that, in terms of effectiveness and efficiency, are significant. And if they are not, change. What's the point of going on with that thing, that diagnosis, that therapy, etc., if it's not taking you anywhere?

MICHAEL: A lot of diagnosis, I think, is just name calling. I've noticed that when therapists use the word "borderline," there is often the word "damn" just before it, like, "Oh, I've got to see that damn borderline at 2:00 o'clock." The diagnoses become insults. "Narcissist" doesn't just mean a person who copes with damaged self-esteem by trying to inflate their worth; "narcissist" is often short-hand for "arrogant pain-in-the-ass."

FLAVIO: How might diagnosis help when seeing someone in brief therapy with, say, so-called "borderline personality disorder"?

MICHAEL: If we said that "borderline" simply means the person tends to see things in black and white, they react very strongly emotionally, and they have chaotic relationships that might give us some ideas of what would be helpful – especially if the person was complaining about being very upset and having chaotic relationships. If they tend to see things in black and white, we can help them learn to see the shades of gray.

I had a client, a woman who was an artist, and she would have qualified for the diagnosis of "borderline." She complained that either you loved her or you hated her, you were her best friend or her worse enemy, everything was good or everything sucked, great to be alive or she ought to kill herself right now. And she was an artist. I got her to go to a store where they sell paint and asked her to bring me 20 different shades of gray, and she brought all these shades of gray and we talked about shades of gray. And then she looked at me and she said, "Is this some kind of metaphor? Are we talking about me?" And I said, "Well, we're talking about shades of gray. And in one way we're talking about color and painting."

FLAVIO: Good!

MICHAEL: Yeah. I said: "It seems like you go from white to black or black to white. What would be halfway, how can you get a little upset or a little angry? Or how could you get hopeful without being completely in love and ready to marry the guy you only met two days ago?" We utilized her artist's sensibility when she would begin to get upset. We were using her vocabulary, her way of experiencing. We met for several months, not just one time. I remember once she came in and she said, "I started to get really angry and I said to myself 'Gray, gray, gray.' Not black, not white, make it gray." And she laughed. So this became a useful metaphor for her. I think the idea of using paint colors came from the borderline diagnosis in some ways. If seeing things in black or white is causing problems, you need to learn the shades of gray. In DBT[34] [dialectical behavior therapy], what they do is teach the person the skills that they need so they would not have the diagnosis. If you could see the shades of gray, not black and white, if you could see that people can be your friend but still sometimes disappoint you so that it's not all good or all bad. You need to learn how to be emotional but not go over-the-top crazy. How are you going to learn emotional regulation? What DBT does, I think, is teach people the skills they need to use so they will no longer qualify for the diagnosis. So, you could use that with all the different diagnoses: what do they need to do so that they will not be a narcissist, etc.? Be interested in other people and how they feel, and not use them to try to fix your self-esteem. What do you need to be able to do so as not to be an official obsessive-compulsive personality? You need to learn how to let go, how to say: "I'll only do it twice and then I'll accept it however it is." It's easy for me to say that here, but you should see me when I'm editing! [laughs] We could think of personality disorder diagnoses as verbs, like borderlining, narcissising, obsessive-compulsing, etc., and then therapy would be about helping people to develop skills to stop borderlining, etc.

FLAVIO: Isn't diagnosis part of clinical expertise?

MICHAEL: The problem with diagnosis to me is that it very quickly becomes "I am The Expert figuring out what's wrong with the client." My expertise becomes "I'm a pathologist" rather than "I'm an expert in bringing out the best in the person." Instead, it's "I'm an expert at finding what's wrong with the person." Most of the books I've read about personality problems and personality disorders have about 250 pages of theory and diagnosis, and then there's a small chapter at the end called "clinical implications" or "therapy."

FLAVIO: This links to the first question, why in many books about brief therapy there isn't a single page about diagnosis? I think I know why, the mainstream perspective of what psychotherapy is, but explaining it might help traditional clinicians to have a different view.

MICHAEL: I think there's a lack for a couple of reasons. One reason is that brief therapists have wanted to show how we are not like those other therapists, and we tend to talk about the other therapists almost like they are evil or bad: "They look for problems. They're negative. They don't have a sense of humor. They're looking for troubles." So it could be good if there were some discussion in brief therapy books of how diagnosis could be helpful in brief therapy.

I think there is also an even bigger issue. Jay Efran, James Hillman (who was a Jungian analyst) and other people have written about it[35]– de Shazer may have talked about this also. We made a mistake in the field of therapy when we decided that we would be like medical doctors, that we will do an assessment that will lead to a diagnosis and that the diagnosis will lead to a treatment. If you think of psychotherapy as a medical treatment, you need a diagnosis. But you can think of therapy as a form of conversation or even a form of theater, like it's a drama and I'm the director. The director doesn't make a diagnosis. The director tries to help the person bring out the performance. "Think about times when you felt a certain way. Who have you ever seen act that way? Imitate them." In some ways it gets right at the heart of what we're doing when we're doing therapy: are we a wise physician sitting there, figuring out what's really wrong?

FLAVIO: I love your answer. I think that is probably a way in which traditional diagnosis could be very helpful for prevention. For example, if I do an assessment that leads to the diagnosis of "Depression" and I know that the prognosis is that 30% of people with this level of depression commit suicide, this could be helpful, maybe even for therapy, but very helpful for prevention. Maybe we can do something in society to prevent suicide in depressed people.

MICHAEL: Sure. If you think the person is depressed, they have lots of the symptoms of depression and (let's make it even worse) maybe they're also drinking a lot of alcohol and they also have a lot of disappointments, like they lost their job, they're getting divorced, their children don't like them and so on, I think it's a reasonable thing to think to yourself, "This person could be at risk for suicide." I don't want to tell them, "You're going to kill yourself," but I think I should ask: "Do you ever think about hurting yourself? When it's bad, what do you think about doing?" And "How do you keep yourself going despite feeling sad?" So, if a diagnosis points to risks, it can help us to be preventive.

I had in my office a woman whose house had caught on fire and had been badly damaged, a couple of hundred thousand dollars worth. It had been a big fire and had ruined part of the house. It had happened about a month before. She reported that before she came in: "For the past three weeks I keep waking up thinking about the fire and what could have happened. We're okay, nobody died and the insurance will pay for the repairs -- but I keep thinking, what if my children had been in the fire? What if we couldn't get out, and will it happen again?"

And she said to me, "Do you think I have post-traumatic stress disorder?" (PTSD) And I said: "No. I think you could develop it. I think right now you are reacting like a normal person to a terrible situation. If you'd told me three weeks ago you had woken up and your house was on fire and you barely got out, but you don't worry about it or even think about it, I would think that's very strange. It's normal that your mind is going over it, partly just to understand it, but also to think about what can you do to prevent it from happening again."

Since she had mentioned PTSD, I got out the book and I said: "Here's what it says for posttraumatic stress disorder. You have to have these things for this amount of time. Do you have seven of the following 11 for more than ..." – you know, whatever the criteria are. And I said, "What do you think you need to do now to prevent getting posttraumatic stress disorder?" And she said, "Well, while I'm thinking about it I need to remember that the danger has passed. I could also call a friend, thank God, maybe read a book." And we went through the list. And so the potential diagnosis gave us some ideas: "You don't want to end up there."

FLAVIO: I see. When you asked the client about the prognosis, actually you helped her to do something to build her prognosis – in a favorable way, of course.

MICHAEL: I hope so. To change the topic a bit, another thought about diagnosis: How do we frame the problem? Do we frame it as an interpersonal problem or do we frame it as an intrapsychic problem? MRI and Jay Haley[36] would look at it interactionally.

Box 6. MRI (Mental Research Institute)

Research and training institute that was based in Palo Alto, California. Founded in 1959 by Don D. Jackson, closed 2019 and now serving as a grant foundation, MRI is one of the originators of interactional/systemic family therapy and the birthplace of Brief Therapy.

*Quotable Quotes

1 "We assume that once one begins to consider that a difficulty is a 'problem,' the continuation, and often the exacerbation of that problem, comes from the formation of a positive feedback system in a closed circuit, which most often revolves around the behaviors of the individuals in the system, intended to solve the difficulty: the original difficulty is the object of an attempt at a 'solution' that intensifies

the original difficulty, and so on" (Weakland, Fisch, Watzlawick, & Bodin, 1974, p. 402).[37]

2. "One of the basic principles of systems theory is that every system is its *own best* explanation [...] What matters to me (exclusively) is the patient's specific problem; and what he has done so far to "solve it," i.e., the *attempted solution*, which in our perspective is the main factor that maintains and exacerbates the problem." (see Watzlawick, Endnote 16 below)

3. "Thus the thrust of therapy is not to get the complainants to do something so much as to stop what they have been doing about the problem [...] In that sense, we would say that we don't treat problems, we treat attempted solutions" (Fisch & Schlanger, 1999, p. 2).

*Key Publications

P. Watzlawick, J.H. Weakland, & R. Fisch (1974). *Change: Principles of Problem Formation and Problem Resolution*. Norton.

R. Fisch, J.H. Weakland, & L. Segal (1982). *The Tactics of Change: Doing Therapy Briefly*. Jossey-Bass.

R. Fisch & K. Schlanger (1999). *Brief Therapy with Intimidating Cases: Changing the Unchangeable*. Jossey-Bass.

P. Watzlawick & J.H. Weakland (Eds.) (1977). *The Interactional View: Studies at the Mental Research Institute, Palo Alto, 1965–1974*. Norton.

It becomes a problem when it impacts other people. Jeff Zeig wrote:

> The way one analyzes a problem often indelibly alters subsequent perceptions. And perceptions determine outcome [...] Treatment follows from diagnostic perceptions.

Similarly, Bill O'Hanlon said:

> I maintain that there are no such 'things' as therapy problems. I think therapists, for the most part, give their clients problems [...] We do not enter therapy neutrally, finding the 'real' problem or problems. We usually only elicit or allow descriptions of problems that fit our theories, that we know how to cope with, make sense of, or solve.[38]

Donald Schon also said:

> Problem setting is a process in which, interactively, we *name* the thing to which we will attend and *frame* the context in which we will attend to them.

So, what diagnostic frame will give us the best way to help them? What's easiest to do?

I used to go to a case conference, and it was like a competition to see who could come up with the worst problem.[39] It would go from reacting to a situation like being nervous when speaking in public to maybe an adjustment disorder to they have a personality disorder to they may have two personality disorders, they have two personality disorders and a learning disorder and maybe A.D.D., etc., etc. It became a contest to show off how much bad stuff could be hypothesized. And then I would raise my hand and say,

> How are we going to help this person? The person only came in because they said they get nervous when they have to talk in public and they want some help with that problem and now we're figuring out everything that possibly could be wrong with them. If we ask enough questions, it's just going to make them more nervous.

So I think we have to be very careful.

FLAVIO: It seems like we're in a loop. We don't want to force people into a diagnosis, into a label, but we recognize that it can be helpful, pointing to roads already traveled. I think that we can come out from this loop connecting to what we said before: it's not that we don't want to use diagnosis, it's that we don't want to take the risk that exists with only *one* kind of diagnosis that forces us to use it even when others could be helpful. It is like wanting to persist in using a fork when other instruments, such as a spoon or chopsticks, can be more suitable. Since *diagnosis* means "through the way of knowledge," we should remember that there are many way*s*.

MICHAEL: The famous psychiatrist Harry Stack Sullivan would ask what I thought was a very interesting question. He would say, "Most people in this situation would do so-and-so. Have you tried that? How did that work?" Maybe they had or had not tried so-and-so, but he was suggesting that before we look for and make more and more complicated problems, let's try commonsense and a simple solution to a problem.[40] If you have somewhat high blood pressure you don't need to start with a heart transplant or maybe even to be put on medicines. Maybe you just need to put less salt on your food and need to drink more water and exercise more – let's try the easy things first. A lot of what we do in brief therapy and SST is help the person to get unstuck. When they begin to solve the problem, other positive things begin happening – they're not so worried, so they get along better with people and because they get along better with people, they have more fun and aren't so depressed and don't stay home and drink. So maybe it goes in a positive direction, an upward "virtuous cycle" instead of a downward "vicious cycle."[41] My dear colleague Bob Rosenbaum used to give an example[42] about somebody coming in with their car seemingly having a lot of problems, and the mechanic examined it and found that there was a little fly stuck in the carburetor and they needed just one thing and everything worked again. They didn't need a new car or a new engine; they just needed, you know, to de-bug one little thing.

FLAVIO: I think: easy things first. I may be opening up a very big door, but a few days ago I was thinking about something like that. It seems to me that many therapists may start with something quite simple, but what happens? It works with one patient and then another, and then with someone else it doesn't. And so the theory becomes more complex, and then more complex.

MICHAEL: If you did the simple thing first and that helps with this one and that one, but there's another person you tried the simple thing with and it doesn't work, then you try another thing. If that doesn't work, then you try yet another thing and if it doesn't work, then maybe with that person you scratch your head and you say, "You know, we tried these simple things but they don't seem to work. What are your ideas? Maybe we should see if there's something else that we should talk about." But don't treat everybody as though they have a personality disorder or a major psychiatric illness that requires years of therapy. I agree with what you're saying, Flavio, about making it harder than it has to be. Most people do not come to therapy wanting a major overhaul. They want help with a particular problem. So try the simple thing first. And if that doesn't work, try another simple thing. And if that doesn't work, then maybe something else.

It's also too much of a burden on the therapist to feel that our job is to be a mastermind like Sherlock Holmes, to be a detective and come up with a brilliant diagnosis and then a brilliant treatment. Our job is mostly to help the client figure out how they can solve a problem. Of course, if somebody could solve their own problem, they would not come to see us. Some people do want some information that we may have that they don't have. I can say, "Well, when don't you have the problem?" or "What's the exception to the problem?" or "How have friends of yours dealt with that problem? Why don't you try that?" But sometimes I will say, "What you're describing, there are therapies that can be helpful for that. Sometimes people do this, sometimes people do that. Would that be interesting?" I think it's tricky because we are experts, we do have lots of psychological knowledge, but we don't want to use our expertise to disempower people.

FLAVIO: I think this is the point: Start simple. Then, if you meet a person with whom the simpler things don't work, you can use more complicated things, but don't forget that with the next person you have to start again with the simple things and not with the complex, complicated things you used with the last person.

MICHAEL: Yes.

FLAVIO: I think I read a chapter by Richard Fisch, in one of your books,[43] and he said that Freud's early therapies were days or weeks, sometimes months. But then they complicated the theory and the therapy started to last many years. I think that it's okay to complicate the theory when you need some more complicated theory and more complicated technique, but if a simpler approach works we should continue to use that for most people.

MICHAEL: When I went to Milwaukee to visit with de Shazer, we went into the room at the Brief Family Therapy Center where they would do the therapy. They had a sign on the wall that said "K.I S.S." It wasn't a poster for the band. It looks like "KISS," but it meant "Keep It Simple, Stupid." Meaning: look for what would be simple and would work rather than make it complicated. They literally had this sign there. There's also another de Shazer story about a sign: people wondered about "K.I.S.S." So somebody put another sign up that said "Simplify, Simplify, Simplify." And de Shazer, when he saw it, went over and he scratched out two of the "Simplify's"!

So this was Occam's Razor, the idea that you should not do with many things what you could do with one thing: keep it simple, stupid. Why don't we see if we can just help the person solve the problem and if it doesn't work then we can ask what are we missing? Is there something else here? But I think what therapists are trained to do, we even have a name for it, "comprehensive assessment." Comprehensive means everything, to comprehend the whole thing. If the person comes in and they say, "Oh, I get nervous when I do X" we may not need to do a comprehensive assessment.

I remember one time a woman came to the clinic in Wisconsin where I was a predoctoral intern a long time ago studying with Carl Whitaker, the family therapist. She was a worrier and was unhappy. I don't even remember what some of the problems were that she was worried about. Carl interviewed her and I sat in the room and watched. He spent almost the whole time asking her,

> Tell me about your family. Oh, how are your children doing? They're getting A's in school —that's wonderful! Oh, tell me about your husband. Oh, he loves you. Do you have friends? Oh, yes – very nice! Where do you live? Oh, wow!

He elicited lots of positive details. After about 30–40 minutes she looked at him and she said, "You know, I really have a good life. I shouldn't worry so much." And he never assessed whether she had Depression or Adjustment Disorder with Depressed Mood or Dysthymia, etc. He just got her to count her blessings, all the things to be grateful for. And by spending enough time on that she brightened up. He also asked her how she would remember all the good things if and when she began to worry.

I once saw a woman who had great anxiety while driving her car, which can be a real problem in the San Francisco Bay area where I live. We started by just sitting in her car. I learned that she was an expert cook – and I love food. When she would begin to drive and start to get nervous, I asked her about her favorite recipes, and she would start describing how to prepare some dish and forget about being anxious. She got over her driving phobia and made me a plate of cookies as a thank you.

FLAVIO: Before we close today let me tell you about a case that reminds me of another example of keeping it simple. A woman came to me for a problem with her anxiety for driving. I started by having her fantasize, you know, having her think about the worst thing, a paradoxical intervention, about driving and then start to try to go in the car, but without driving. And in the second session I said, "Okay, now take your car and drive a little, you know, just for 50 meters." In the third session I said, "Now drive around your building and then just around the block." And then she said, "Yes, it's going very well. I just think I need to have more confidence, start to drive in traffic, but I need someone else with me." And I said, "Okay, so stop the therapy, go in a driving school, and do some driving with a driving schoolteacher." So she stopped therapy and went to take some drives with a professional driving teacher. Two months ago she called me and said: "I'm driving all alone and it is going very well. This summer I will go for a road trip with my car. Thank you for helping me, and thank you for saving me money" because the driving teacher does not cost as much as therapy!

MICHAEL: [*laughs*] That was real practical. You helped her solve her problem.

FLAVIO: Yeah. She just needed to do some driving lessons.

MICHAEL: That was very good. You encouraged her and helped her feel ready and that she could do it. But if you had looked in a therapy book and given her a diagnosis, they would have told you she needs 10 or 15 sessions to learn new ways of breathing and she needed to learn mental imagery and she needed to find out where the underlying maladaptive schemas came from and what childhood trauma she was repressing and what she was avoiding in her current life for her secondary gain. She'd still be your patient.

There is the brief therapy technique of prescribing the symptom, like paradoxically advising a client to make themselves have a panic attack so they can see that they have control and that they can survive being anxious. There's also a phrase in English, "fake it until you make it," meaning act "as if" you don't have so much anxiety even if you do. Pretend you don't. I know a married couple and once when they were having communication problems and the man was being very critical, they went to therapy and the therapist said to the man, "Who's your favorite movie star?" and he named a charming, debonair fellow. And the therapist said, "Why do you like him?" "Oh, because he's handsome and he's articulate and he's kind and he always gets the girl at the end." And the therapist said, "How would this movie star talk to your wife?" and the man explained how he imagined the star would act and what he would say to her. And the therapist said, "Why don't you pretend you're the movie star and, for the next week, when you begin to have a conflict, act like you're him?" And the guy said, "Well, but..." and the therapist said, "You know, just try it" and the wife laughed and then the therapist reminded him that the star gets the girl in the end. And it worked – he tried it and when he acted nicer the wife responded differently and they got unstuck and things got better. Now the reason I know about this case is because I was the husband – not the therapist! Otherwise we could still be writing our check and going every week and talking about male and female roles and communication styles and our childhoods and family-of-origin intergenerational dynamics.

FLAVIO: That's funny!

MICHAEL: Therapists often find some way to make it more complicated rather than getting to a solution.

I want to say one other thing very quickly. When young therapists begin their training, they oftentimes work in a clinic or in a hospital and they see the worst, most difficult patients. They've been patients for many years, they've been in and out of hospitals and they've tried to kill themselves. They're very heavy, serious and discouraging cases. What that does is it often teaches the neophyte therapist that patients don't get better. They have too many problems. It's too heavy. There's always another problem behind this one. If you were going to medical school, you would not start by doing open heart surgery or replacing people's hips or their knees – you would start by taking their temperature, giving a shot and dealing with little problems. Well, I think what happens when we get too trained into diagnosis is we begin to think about everything that could be wrong. Sometimes we do need to know that, but a lot of times we don't. I think it would be better to look for some more good things about the person. "Tell me something else. What do you like about this person? What might be hopeful about this person?" Maybe when looking to the past, we should spend more time looking for the happiness.[44] I think that's the opposite of diagnosing, at least how most diagnosis is used.

We'll be talking more soon, my friend – we need to figure out our schedule. Do you have a last word for today?

FLAVIO: My last word is: keep it simple.

Box 7. Chapter 2 Summary: Diagnosis and Brief Therapy

The word *diagnosis* comes from Greek and Latin words meaning "the way of knowledge," so a useful diagnosis should give information that points the way to help the client. Brief therapists often don't use conventional forms of diagnosis. Knowing a *DSM* diagnosis does not specify how to help a particular client. Productive versus pejorative diagnosis and different ways of doing diagnosis are explored with clinical examples. Information is also provided about Steve de Shazer, Jay Haley, and the strategic-interactional approach of the Mental Research Institute (MRI).

Reflection Question: Describe a time when a diagnosis misled you.

Notes

1 See M.F. Hoyt (1995). *Brief Therapy and Managed Care* (p. 257). Jossey-Bass.

2 Frances (2013, p. 12) said that "All of our diagnoses are now based on subjective judgments that are inherently fallible and prey to capricious change." A. Frances (2013). *Saving Normal: An Insider's Revolt Against Out-of-Control Psychiatric Diagnosis, DSM-5, Big Pharma and the Medicalization of Ordinary Life*. William Morrow.

3 See "On the Importance of Keeping It Simple and Taking the Patient Seriously: A Conversation with Steve de Shazer and John Weakland." In M.F. Hoyt. *Interviews with Brief Therapy Experts* (pp. 1–33). Brunner-Routledge.

4 Quoted in J.K. Zeig (Ed.) (1980). *A Teaching Seminar with Milton H. Erickson, M.D.* Brunner/Mazel. The father of modern medical education, Sir William Osler, (quoted in Sacks, 1995, p. vii) also said: "Ask not what disease the person has, but rather what person the disease has." O. Sacks (1995). *An Anthropologist on Mars: Seven Paradoxical Tales*. Random House.

5 See S. Beer (1970). "Managing Modern Complexity." *Futures*, 2(3), 245–257; and P. Watzlawick, "'Insight' May Cause Blindness." In J.K. Zeig (Ed.), *The Evolution of Psychotherapy: The Third Conference* (pp. 309–317). Brunner/Mazel.

6 K. Tomm (1990). "A Critique of the DSM." *Dulwich Centre Newsletter, 3*, 5–8. Also see J. Hargens & U. Grau (1994). "Meta-Dialogue." *Contemporary Family Therapy, 16*(6), 451–462.

7 J.K. Simon & T.S. Nelson (2007). *"I Am More than My Label": Solution-Focused Brief Therapy Practice with Long-Term Users of Mental-Health Services*. Haworth Press.

8 I.D. Yalom (2002). *The Gift of Therapy*. HarperCollins. See p. 4.

9 J.A. Lieberman (2015). *Shrinks: The Untold Story of Psychiatry*. Brown, Little.

10 A. Bierce (1957). *The Devil's Dictionary* (p. 36). Sagamore Press [work originally published 1906].

11 See "Solution Building and Language Games: A Conversation with Steve de Shazer (and Some After Words with Insoo Kim Berg)." In M.F. Hoyt (2001). *Interviews with Brief Therapy Experts* (pp. 158–183). Brunner-Routledge.

12 See P. Watzlawick, J.B. Baveles, & D.D. Jackson (1967). *Pragmatics of Human Communication: A Study of Interactional Patterns, Pathologies, and Paradoxes*. Norton. Also: G. Nardone & C. Portelli (2005). *Knowing Through Changing: The Evolution of Brief Strategic Therapy*. Crown House Publishing; and G. Vitry, C. de Scorraille, C. Portelli, & M.F. Hoyt (2021). "Redundant Attempted Solutions: Operative Diagnoses and Strategic Interventions to Disrupt More of the Same." *Journal of Systemic Therapies, 40*(4), 11–28.

13 As Nardone and Valteroni (2017/2020, p. 6, emphases in original) put it: "It is the solution that has proven effective in *solving* the problem that *explains* the inner workings of the problem itself." G. Nardone & E. Valteroni (2020). *Advanced Brief Strategic Therapy for Young People with Anorexia Nervosa: An Effective Guide for Clinicians*. Routledge (work first published in Italian in 2017).

14 See M.F. Hoyt (2001). "The Squeaky Wheel: Don't Let Managed Care Shortchange Your Clients." *Family Therapy Networker, 25*(1), 19–20. Reprinted in M.F. Hoyt, *The Present is a Gift: Mo' Better Stories from the World of Brief Therapy* (pp. 126–129). iUniverse. Also see M.F. Hoyt (2000), "Likely Future Trends and Attendant Ethical Concerns Regarding Managed Mental Health Care." In *Some Stories Are Better than Others* (pp. 77–108). Brunner/Mazel; and M.F. Hoyt & S. Friedman (2000). "Dilemmas of Postmodern Practice under Managed Care and Some Pragmatics for Increasing the Likelihood of Treatment Authorization." In M.F. Hoyt, *Some Stories Are Better Than Others* (pp. 109–117). Brunner/Mazel.

15 In New York City in August 1998. See M.F. Hoyt, S.D. Miller, B.S. Held, & W.J. Matthews (2000). "About Constructivism (Or, If Four Colleagues Talked in New

York, Would Anyone Hear It?)." *Journal of Systemic Therapies*, 2000, *19*(4), 76–92. Reprinted in M.F. Hoyt (2001). *Interviews with Brief Therapy Experts* (pp. 206–225). Brunner-Routledge. Also see B.S. Held (1992). "The Problem of Strategy within the Systemic Therapies." *Journal of Marital and Family Therapy*, *18*, 25–34; and B.S. Held (1995). *Back to Reality: A Critique of Postmodern Theory in Psychotherapy.* Norton.

16 "Constructing Therapeutic Realities: A Conversation with Paul Watzlawick." In M.F. Hoyt (2001). *Interviews with Brief Therapy Experts* (pp. 144–157). Brunner-Routledge.

17 Thus, Yuval Noah Harari (2015, p. 238) explains:

> What is the difference between describing 'how' and explaining 'why'? To describe 'how' means to reconstruct the series of specific events that led from one point to another. To explain 'why' means to find causal connections that account for the occurrence of this particular series of events to the exclusion of all others.

See Y.N. Harari (2015). *Sapiens: A Brief History of Humankind.* HarperCollins.

18 B. Wampold & Z.G. Imel (2015). *The Great Psychotherapy Debate: The Evidence for What Makes Psychotherapy Work* (2nd ed.). Routledge.

19 See F. Cannistrá (2019). "A Violent Life: Using Brief Therapy 'Logics' to Facilitate Change." In M.F. Hoyt & M. Bobele (Eds.), *Creative Therapy in Challenging Situations* (pp. 47–57). Routledge. Also see Chapter 7, this volume.

20 See P. Watzlawick, J.H. Weakland, & R. Fisch (1974). *Change: Principles of Problem Formation and Problem Resolution.* Norton; R. Fisch, J.H. Weakland, & L. Segal (1982). *The Tactics of Change: Doing Therapy Briefly.* Jossey-Bass; R. Fisch & K. Schlanger (1999). *Brief Therapy with Intimidating Cases: Changing the Unchangeable.* Jossey-Bass; S. de Shazer (1988). *Clues: Investigating Solutions in Brief Therapy.* Norton.

21 At a 1995 meeting of leading strategic therapists, Jay Haley said (and John Weakland concurred):

> I would like to see this group be more radical and do something that others probably wouldn't do. Since, for example, the *DSM-IV* is only individual, I think this group should make a *therapy DSM* in which the basic unit is two people and you formulate problems in a way that is helpful to a therapist. Instead of calling a kid a 'school phobia' you call him a 'school avoidance problem.' That guides you to do something. It also guides you to think about why he is avoiding school. It would be interesting as a task to make a diagnostic manual that is for therapists, not for the institutions and insurance companies and so on (who might never accept it). But it would be very good for training, because you would begin to find symptoms falling out in terms of certain ways to deal with them in order to get people over them.

See M.F. Hoyt (2000). "Unmuddying the Waters: A 'Common Ground' Conference." In *Some Stories Are Better Than Others: Doing What Works in Brief Therapy and Managed Care* (pp. 195–200). Brunner/Mazel.

22 G. Bateson, D.D. Jackson, J. Haley, & J.H. Weakland (1956). "Toward a Theory of Schizophrenia." *Behavioral Science*, *1*, 251–264.

23 Back cover endorsement of M. Talmon (1993). *Single Session Solutions: A Guide to Practical, Effective, and Affordable Therapy.* Addison-Wesley.

24 For more on single-session therapy, see M. Talmon (1990). *Single-Session Therapy: Maximizing the Effect of the First (and Often Only) Therapeutic Encounter.* Jossey-Bass; M.F. Hoyt & M. Talmon (Eds.) (2014). *Capturing the Moment.* Crown House Publishing; M.F. Hoyt et al. (Eds.) (2018). *Single-Session Therapy by Walk-in or Appointment.* Routledge; F. Cannistrà & F. Piccirilli (Eds.) (2018). *Terapia a Seduta Singola.* Giunti; M.F. Hoyt et al. (Eds.) (2021). *Single Session Thinking and Practice in Global, Cultural, and Familial Contexts: Expanding Applications.* Routledge;

W. Dryden (2017). *Single-Session Integrated CBT (SSI-CBT)*. Routledge; W. Dryden (2019). *Single-Session Therapy: 100 Key Points and Techniques*. Routledge; and M.F. Hoyt & F. Cannistrà (Chapters 6 and 8, this volume).

25 These ideas are developed further in F. Cannistrà (2021). "The Vital Role of the Therapist's Mindset." In M.F. Hoyt, J. Young, & P. Rycroft (Eds.), *Single Session Thinking and Practice in Global, Cultural, and Familial Contexts: Expanding Applications* (pp. 77–88). Routledge; and in Chapter 3 this volume.

26 See B.E. Wampold (2015). "How Important Are the Common Factors in Psychotherapy? An Update." *World Psychiatry*, 14(3), 270–277.

27 "For creativity to be real, it must be a genuine *process* of undetermined becoming: it cannot be the mere unfolding of an already completely determined sequence of steps to a ready-made conclusion." G.S. Morson (1994). *Narrative and Freedom: The Shadows of Time*. Yale University Press.

28 F. Cannistrà (2019). "A Violent Life: Using Brief Therapy 'Logics' to Facilitate Change." In M.F. Hoyt & M. Bobele (Eds.), *Creative Therapy in Challenging Situations Unusual Interventions to Help Clients* (pp. 47–57). Routledge.

29 For discussion of client/patient, see Note 1 on page 23 of this volume.

30 J. Young (2018). "Single-Session Therapy: The Misunderstood Gift That Keeps on Giving." In M.F. Hoyt et al. (Eds.), *Single-Session Therapy by Walk-in or Appointment* (pp. 40–58). Routledge.

31 M.F. Hoyt (1989). "Psychodiagnosis of Personality Disorders." *Transactional Analysis Journal*, 19, 101–113. Reprinted in *Brief Therapy and Managed Care* (pp. 257–279). Jossey-Bass, 1995.

32 M.F. Hoyt (2001, p. 11). "On the Importance of Keeping It Simple and Taking the Patient Seriously: A Conversation with Steve de Shazer and John Weakland." In M.F. Hoyt (Ed.), *Interviews with Brief Therapy Experts* (pp. 1–33). Brunner-Routledge.

33 L. Hoffman (1990). "Constructing Realities: An Art of Lenses." *Family Process*, 29, 1–12; M.A. Hubble & W.H. O'Hanlon (1992). "Theory Countertransference." *Dulwich Centre Newsletter*, 1, 25–30.

34 See M.M. Linehan (2015). *DBT Skills Training Manual* (2nd ed.). Guilford Press.

35 See J.S. Efran & M. Greene (2005). "The Art of Therapeutic Conversation." *Psychotherapy Networker*, 29(6), 35–36; and J. Hillman (1996). *The Soul's Code: In Search of Character and Calling*. Random House.

36 Also see J.K. Zeig (1988). "Foreword." In E. Bader & P.T. Pearson (pp. vii–ix), *In Quest of the Mythical Mate: Developmental Approach to Diagnosis and Treatment in Couples Therapy*. Brunner/Mazel; B. O'Hanlon (1999). *Evolving Possibilities: Selected Papers of Bill O'Hanlon* (S. O'Hanlon & B. Bertolino, Eds.; p. 148). Brunner/Mazel; D. Schon (1983). *The Reflective Practitioner: How Professionals Think in Action* (pp. 39–42). Basic Books.

37 J.H. Weakland, R. Fisch, P. Watzlawick, & A. Bodin (1974). "Brief Therapy: Focused Problem Resolution." *Family Process*, 13(2), 141–168.

38 Michael added later: I recall Bill pointing out the artificiality of diagnosis, quipping that "They've done thousands of autopsies, and they have never found 'a borderline'!"

39 See P. Meehl (1973). "Why I Do Not Attend Case Conferences." In *Psychodiagnosis: Selected Papers*. University of Minnesota Press.

40 H.S. Sullivan (1954): "I think the development of psychiatric skill consists in very considerable measure of doing a lot with very little – making a rather precise move which has a high probability of achieving what you're attempting to achieve with a minimum of time and words." *The Psychiatric Interview*. Norton.

41 P. Wender (1968). "Vicious and Virtuous Cycles: The Role of Deviation-Amplifying Feedback in the Origin and Perpetuation of Behavior." *Psychiatry*, 31, 309–324.

42 R. Rosenbaum, M.F. Hoyt, & M. Talmon (1990). "The Challenge of Single-Session Therapies: Creating Pivotal Moments." In R.A. Wells & V.J. Giannetti (Eds.), *Handbook of the Brief Psychotherapies* (pp. 165–189). Plenum. Reprinted in M.F. Hoyt (1995). *Brief Therapy and Managed Care* (pp. 105–139). Jossey-Bass.

43 See R. Fisch (1994). "Basic Elements in the Brief Therapies." In M.F. Hoyt (Ed.), *Constructive Therapies* (pp. 126–139). Guilford Press.

44 See S.D. Miller (1992). "The Symptoms of Solution." *Journal of Strategic and Systemic Therapies, 11,* 1–11.

Chapter 3

Mindset in Brief Therapy

FLAVIO: Let's talk about the *mindset*.

MICHAEL: About what?

FLAVIO: The mindset. We were talking about it in the last few days. Let's talk about that in a more general way, I mean, how important is the mindset for doing a brief therapy? In the last decades, many authors have focused themselves on techniques, on protocols, on evocative language and on communication, but it seems to me that few of them spend much time talking about the underlying mindset. For example, if you don't enter into a brief therapy mindset or if you don't think that a single session or a few sessions are OK, you simply can't help the person in a single step.

MICHAEL: For me the *mindset* is how you set your mind, how you approach or what you believe – your orientation, your expectation, your hope, what you think is possible. *Mindset* refers to a set of beliefs that influence how you think, feel and behave in any given situation.[1]

And so the mindset with single session is, "We could get something done today that would be good. And maybe one session is all the person needs." In brief therapy, we may not think it will happen today, but it will happen soon. At least we don't have to think about "a long time" or "it goes slow." When I asked Jay Haley why they called it "Brief Therapy," he said it was mostly to distinguish it from the expectation that therapy would be long – which was the dominant psychodynamic view at that time.[2]

I think a term close to *mindset* is *expectation* or *hope*. A famous person once said, "If you think somebody is going to be a success, or if you think they're going to be a failure, you're probably right." If you think success, they will have success. And if you think failure, they will have failure. When you sit down with a client and you say, "Let's see what we can get done today, maybe we'll have enough time. We'll do enough. We may only need to meet once. Are you interested in that?" they may go, "Well, yeah, if we can." But if you say, "Well, we're going to start today, but this will take a long time and we will have to get to know one another and you will have to come back many times and we will go slow," then the person thinks, "Well, not too much will happen today."

DOI: 10.4324/9781003307709-4

FLAVIO: It's a theory problem – don't you agree?

MICHAEL: Part of it is the theory. If your theory is, "We have to slowly develop a relationship. We have to slowly uncover the problems. We have to slowly talk about them so we don't stimulate resistance or make a trauma or make it too difficult. Slowly, slowly, go slowly," then our theory is telling us the speed at which we can go. If our theory says, "People make changes when they are ready, and sometimes they can make a change quickly, or almost in the moment, or in the moment," then our theory allows us to be open to the possibility that change will happen NOW. So there's a joke I sometimes tell when I'm teaching. There was a famous American baseball player, his name was Yogi Berra, and he was famous because he would say things that were very clever but he would sound like he did not know what he had said – but they were very wise. One time someone asked him, "What time is it?" and he said, "Do you mean NOW?" Meaning *in the present*. Meaning that *there's only the present* or *the present is a gift*. (That's the title of a book that I once published![3])

FLAVIO: Why is it so difficult for many…?

MICHAEL: So, I think the reason therapy became longer is because of several things. One is the theory, but another is many problems do not get all better in one visit. It takes time, the person gets some ideas, they have to think about it, they have to practice, the social situation may not be conducive. Maybe it brings up another problem.

Another reason why it takes longer is money. The therapist wants to be paid and so I want you to come back so we can keep talking. That often influences it. Another reason why therapy takes longer is that when Freud was beginning to develop psychoanalysis, psychoanalysis was partially a therapeutic tool to try to help people. But it also was a research instrument, like a microscope to look at things. And they discovered that if the therapist did not talk very much, the patient would begin to project ideas onto the therapist: "You're like my mother, you're like my father, you're like my brother and my sister." The transference would happen. They also found early on that if the therapist did not do too much, the conversation would go from talking about facts to more unconscious ideas, bigger patterns and beliefs that the person had not thought much about. So, therapy became longer and longer because they said, "This is interesting: if we don't do much, if we're passive or quiet, a blank screen, wow, look what happens! They begin to relate to us like we're their parents. They begin to have memories about different things."

FLAVIO: They confused therapy with analysis.

MICHAEL: Exactly. So, in 1937, I think it was '37, Sigmund Freud wrote his last great paper. It was called *Analysis: Terminable and Interminable*. "Terminable and interminable." They could have called it "Analysis, Finite or Infinite" or "Time-Limited or Forever." He said, analysis goes on and on and you can always analyze – but it doesn't always help people.

So he said in the paper, he said it in German, but I'll paraphrase it in English:

> We need to develop a more durable, strong, efficient, therapeutic tool to help people more quickly. We could use some of the ideas of analysis, but we also have to use not just 'insight' but also suggestion, guidance, education, encouragement. We have to try to help the person get better quicker. When we do that, we are no longer doing analysis. We're not just blank and let's see what happens. But people come for help. They don't come just to be a research subject.

And so, in his last major paper, he said, analysis is too slow. It's interminable. It goes on forever. So let's use different techniques. Freud himself, I understand, sometimes would give people advice. He would talk with them. He did not just listen to them.

FLAVIO: Like the single-session Freud case I sent you – it's very interesting.

MICHAEL: Yes – she had been a girl when she met Freud. What happened?

FLAVIO: In that case, the client, a very young girl, she was 12 I think, or 14, I don't remember, her father brought her to Sigmund Freud and she said that Freud just listened to her for 10 minutes, 20 minutes, 30 minutes, not so long, and then he just gave her advice: "You should be nice with your father," because it was in the early 20th century, but he also told her, "You have to be yourself, you have to find your way to do things, so be nice and find your way to do things." She said that the single session changed her life. He didn't do psychoanalysis. It was not analysis, it was single-session psychological counseling.[4]

MICHAEL: He did not interpret her unconscious conflict. It sounds like he said, "Use your energy to think about who you want to be in your life. Become your own person, choose what you want to do."

FLAVIO: And I can imagine that someone can say, "Yes, but that's not psychopathology. With a real psychopathology you have to do something different, you have to do psychoanalysis" – but in this way of thinking for me there is an error, a mistake. The mistake, the error is that we think that "psychopathology" is a thing, a concrete thing, and that you can distinguish between psychopathology and non-psychopathology, and simple problems.

MICHAEL: They can say that if the person changes quickly, it wasn't a real pathology. If they don't change, then it's pathology. But, you know, if she had gone to a different doctor, they could have said she's anti-social, anti-authoritarian. Now we might say she has oppositional defiant disorder. Maybe she wasn't terrible. She wasn't taking lots of drugs and cutting her wrists and doing really bad things, but he intervened in a way that helped her realize that she wanted to be in charge of herself in a good way.

FLAVIO: I told you before about the case of the binge eater. Her life was a mess: binge eater, depressive, she took lots of medications and her mother had died 3 weeks before. And in just one session – we stopped in an unplanned way because she lost her job – but in that session she followed the suggestions and most importantly she probably found something that helped her to enhance her resources in that moment, and she solved the problem. Four months later she was OK. I sent her an email to check how she was and she said she was fine, she was happy and she had no binges in 4 months. I don't think that this means that all binge eaters can do that, but some can.

MICHAEL: But some can, and at least one did. And more than one. I have known such people in my office. A young woman came once, she was 19 or 20 years old. Her mother had said, "You go talk to the doctor." I said, "Why?" She said, "My mother's worried because sometimes I eat a lot and I make myself throw up." And I said, "Do you also starve?" She said, "No." I said, "You know about anorexia?" She said, "I know, but I'm not anorexic, but sometimes I start to be bulimic. I binge and I purge." I said, "How long have you been doing it?" She said, "Oh, maybe six months." "Everyday?" "Not everyday. A couple of times a week, I do it." I said to her,

> You are at a very important point and it is very nice to meet you here today in my office. You're standing at a fork in the road, and if you go down this path, it's going to get worse and worse. You will lose control. You will be doing it more. Throwing up will ruin your throat, will ruin your teeth, will ruin your digestion, your chemistry, your body. You will risk becoming a crazy, unhappy person. Or you will say, 'I'm going to go the other way. I still feel sometimes that I want to do it, but I have to find a better way, when I feel stressed, not to do this.' And you are standing at the fork in the road. Do not decide yet which way you want to go, because if you go to the way where you throw up, it may feel good for a little while. You know, keep your weight down. You can eat all you want. When you're upset, you can do this and forget what your problems are. It will be good for a few months. And then you'll get sick and ruin your life. Or you can go the other way and it will be hard for a few months, and maybe very difficult, because it's becoming a habit. So, what do you want to do? You're about to make a big decision that will change your life. I'm a doctor, so of course I want you to be healthy, but I think you'll have to decide, maybe today, maybe not, but the longer you wait, the harder it is and I can tell because I've seen a lot of people faced with this decision: You are at the point where today would be a good day to make the decision. What do you want to do?

We talked, and she said, "I don't want to do that." I said, "But you have been doing that. Do you really want to do that?" She said, "Well,

I did that, but I don't think I should do that." I said, "Why not?" She said, "Well, you know, you told me I'll get sick." I said, "Yeah, you'll get sick. You'll be in a rehabilitation psych unit. Your breath will smell like vomit, and it will be on your clothes. You'll be crazy. Your hair will fall out and you'll stop having your menstrual cycle. You'll be crazy. Your friends won't like you anymore – but hey, why not?

She laughed and she said, "You're a good salesman!" And I said, "Only if you want to buy it. I'm a very good salesman, when somebody is smart enough to know what I'm talking about, that I might be right." I said, "You know, I will be glad to meet with you again and again if we have to -- but everything that we're going to talk about, we've talked about in the last 10 minutes, the last 20 minutes. We can talk about other things in your life, school, boys, the future or your parents, whatever, but sooner or later you have to make a decision. Is this the way you want to live your life?

And she said, "But what if it's hard? I think it's going to be very hard." I said, "Of course it's going to be hard. If, if you were starting to drink too much, and I said, 'Do you want to be an alcoholic? You know, it'll be fun. You'll party and then your liver will be ruined, and maybe boys will rape you, and you will be a drunk, and you'll be stupid, and you won't have a job, and your skin will look ugly because you don't take care of yourself. Would you want to be an alcoholic?'

She said, "No." I said, "Well, you're like an alcoholic with food and now you have to decide." And we had the one meeting. She said, "I don't think I need to come back." I said, "Wonderful. Will you call me in a couple of weeks and tell me, I really want to know how you are and what you decide."

She called me and then she even called me again in a couple of months: "I stopped doing that. I'm better." This was one session. Now somebody else I could have said the same thing to her and she might have said "Go to hell" or "I'll think about it." But I think she was ready. She wanted to change. It wasn't too difficult for her – it was difficult, but not too difficult. Maybe I'm not an expert, but my experience with people with the beginning of an eating disorder is either they get better quickly or it's often a long, long process. Most of the books make it sound like it's always a long process and sometimes it is, but I had a feeling she would be able to change more quickly.

FLAVIO: You blocked her unsuccessful attempt, but you didn't assume the worse.

MICHAEL: Right.

The other thing I wanted to say is therapists do not fix patients. We do not change patients. We do not cure patients. We do not resolve psychopathology. We don't work miracles. What we do is create the conditions where patients decide to fix themselves, help themselves, work a miracle, cure themselves, resolve their problem, no longer have the problem, don't do that anymore. Even Milton Erickson said that it is the patient who does all the work.[5] The therapist provides the weather, though, the wind and the sun. We provide the context and encouragement. But the only way I could stop somebody from bingeing would be if I would follow them around and grab their hand and not let them eat, not let them put the food in their mouth. Then I could stop them from bingeing, for a few minutes. The only way I could stop somebody from being depressed would be if every time they started to get depressed, I shook them and maybe told jokes. I don't know what it would be. I think it's important to realize, to use my golf metaphor, that we are the caddy and not the player and our job is to be such a good caddy that the player plays well.[6] A good caddy says, "Be careful on the left, there is water. Be careful on the right, there's your mother. Be careful in front, there's sand." So you guide them, but it has to come from the client. When something gets better, when somebody gets better, we sometimes say, "I did it, I cured Mrs. Esposito of her panic disorder. I fixed her." Well, we did not really cure her.[7] She cured herself, if you want to use the word "cure," or she decided herself to do something different. We never cure people. This gets at the idea of who has the power, who really has the control. Some people – Salvador Minuchin, Milton Erickson and Bob Goulding come to mind – they were so good at talking to people that the person would think, "I can do it. I can do it." *"Sí, se puede"* *en español* – "Yes, I can." *Sí, se puede.* "I can do it."[8] That is the art of therapy. The therapist is like a director in a theatre, and we're trying to get a brilliant performance from the actor.

Okay, we're now turning south, to stay on Highway 101 South. Otherwise we would be going into downtown San Luis Obispo. It's a nice town. There's a university there, but we don't need to go there today.

FLAVIO: What is the name of the city?

MICHAEL: This town? San Luis Obispo. In California, the Spanish created missions, *las misiónes*, up and down the state, so many of the old towns have Spanish names.

FLAVIO: It's interesting. I see a parallelism to what you just said, what you were just talking about.

MICHAEL: Not going to places that might be interesting but will take us out of our way?

FLAVIO: Exactly. I read that in California when the Christian priests came and started the missions they went around and said to the Native Americans, "You have to change your faith, because I have the truth, your faith is wrong."

MICHAEL: Right. So one reason therapy sometimes takes so long is, "I have to get you to stop being who you are and start to get you to believe in my beliefs, my psychotherapy religion, my culture." It's a detour.

FLAVIO: I don't necessarily want to say that the other therapists are like the Christians with the Natives, I don't want to quite say that, but I want to say that it's interesting the conflict and the opposition you can create, that you can build in people, if you try and impose your way to see things, if you want to try to "educate" them your way.

MICHAEL: In Narrative Therapy, they have a very good term. They talk about *colonization,*[9] where you get colonized.

> So, who convinced you to believe that? How were you recruited to think that way? Why do you believe that people of your group are not good, or women are not as smart or it is wrong to be attracted to men instead of women or women instead of men, or why you're not supposed to go to college or why you're not...

People have beliefs that they learn, included beliefs that sometimes make them sick. There are other reasons, too, but colonization is one.

FLAVIO: That reminds me that millions of people were "treated" with a stroke of the pen when *DSM-III* cancelled homosexuality from the list of mental illnesses.

MICHAEL: Exactly. A lot of brief therapy tries to work with the clients' own belief systems to help them be a better version of themselves, instead of saying "You have to learn a whole different way of being." Now, if the person was indoctrinated or inculcated or brainwashed into a belief system that limits them, then Narrative Therapy says, "Is that the way you want to think about yourself, your preference, or is that the way people tell you to think about yourself? How would you like to feel? How would you like to see things?" Most people, when they're asked, will say: "I would like to think I'm an intelligent person" or "I'm a good person" or "There's nothing wrong with me." So it's trying to give the person a sense of empowerment.

When we talk about mindset, in brief therapy and single session therapy, we say there are three elements.[10] One is the *expectation* that you can make changes. A second is *empowerment,* helping the person see they have power, they are competent, they have choice, they have control, they have autonomy, they have responsibility, they have individuality and they have the right to do what they want to do as long as they don't hurt somebody else. So that's empowerment. It's kind of a funny thing to say, "We empower somebody." How do we give them the power? It's more we show them that they have the power and we don't take it away from them. We ask them questions to remind them that they have choices. What do they want? "Do you like chocolate or do you like vanilla? How do you know you like chocolate?" So, one aspect of the mindset is the expectation that something good could happen. Two is empowerment. And three is the idea of *time, il tempo,* the present time, NOW. So, when are you going to do it? Tomorrow? Yesterday? Remember when we were driving and we saw the elephant seals and we said, "Oh, that's cool." We went by and I was thinking, "Oh, we'll see them someday." Then you said, "How about now?" And we turned around. We went to look at them. We had a different experience. That was saying, we can do something in the moment – even though now we're only talking about sightseeing – but it's the same idea that there really is no time but the present. The future is someday. The past is yesterday... or, as I heard someone say, "The past is history. Tomorrow's a mystery. Today is a gift. That's why we call it the present." The idea is that somebody can really do something different. Right now. There comes some moment where the person says, "No, I'm not going to get drunk again," or "No, I'm not going to go with that bad person again," or "No, I'm not going to be a jerk and fight with everybody. I'm angry, but that doesn't help. I'm going to do something different." And that is the moment, the moment of truth, the moment of change. That's the moment where life *is*, the present. It's not the past and it's not the future. The only time people ever change is in the present. You can't go back and change what happened when you were a child. You can think about it differently and be in charge of it rather than it being in charge of you, but unless you're under age 18, you're not really going to have a different childhood. And I can't really change what hasn't happened yet. *Therapy doesn't help people have a different past – it helps people have a different future.* It's very difficult for people to accept that all the things that have happened are maybe now in their mind, and they can influence us – but still there's a moment where I could do something different.

FLAVIO: We see that, but often we as therapists we have to see problems. I remember I used to study to become a Jungian therapist and then I discovered strategic therapy.

MICHAEL: That's what happened to Watzlawick. He said that when he was a Jungian analyst he knew almost everything about Siberian creation myths, but it bothered him that he didn't know what to do with a person who chewed his fingernails.[11]

FLAVIO: In the very first moment I was like, yes, I will probably use strategic therapy just to fix the symptoms and I will continue with Jungian analysis, because it was difficult to me to abandon a paradigm, the Jungian paradigm, the psychoanalytic paradigm that I had studied for so many years. And then I completed brief strategic therapy and abandoned the Jungian therapy and actually never did a single Jungian therapy. I had already studied solution-focused brief therapy [SFBT] a bit many years before, but a few months ago when I went to London for SFBT training it was at first terrible for me because I was a strategic therapist, and as a strategic therapist, techniques do matter to me a lot and in London I was introduced in a new paradigm in which you must not give techniques to the client and you only use questions and solution talk, and the client does most of the work.

MICHAEL: Whose therapy is it? It's the client's therapy! Whose life is it? It's the client's life!

FLAVIO: Yes, it's very difficult for us as therapists to leave our models, to leave our paradigms. It shouldn't be so difficult, because, ok, maybe you are a psychodynamic therapist or a strategic therapist or whatever, but you are a therapist, first of all, and you should probably put yourself in a mindset that allows you to help the client in the best possible way. You shouldn't put yourself in the mindset of embracing a theory like a faith: "I believe in attachment theory, I believe in conflict therapy." They are constructs, they aren't things, they are ideas and you need to use those ideas but not believe that they are absolute truths.

MICHAEL: I went to the first Evolution of Psychotherapy conference in 1985 in Phoenix, Arizona. It doesn't usually snow in Arizona, and the first day it snowed, which was sort of like a signal from the heavens: "Something special is about to happen. Pay attention." So, I went to hear the first speaker and they were brilliant and I had read many of their books. Yes, yes, yes. And then I went to hear the second speaker and they were brilliant and I had read many of their books – yes, yes, yes – and then they said, "The first speaker is wrong. I am right." Then the third speaker spoke and said, "They're both nice, but I am more right," and then the fourth, you know, and by the end of the day, I was crazy – and free. Like, "Oh, what am I going to do? All these things that I thought were true, our theories, are constructions that are useful to think about if they help, but they're only ideas." It was like my mind was falling out onto the floor: "I can't believe I didn't know that none of this is true. It's all ideas." And lots are good ideas. Sometimes they've been very good, but if the idea gets in the way, I may need another idea, instead of saying the patient is the problem if the theory or the idea doesn't give me a good way to help this person. I was trained in one school of therapy, learned it very well. I liked it, knew a lot about it. It was famous. It was very intellectually satisfying. But then I learned something, and then something else. But then I felt like maybe I'm being disloyal, I'm cheating. So I think this is a big problem, when we have schools of therapy. In English we say, "fish swim in a school." Yes, there's cognitive-behavioral and psychodynamic and attachment and they are all good for something and some are better than others. You can use different ideas. We need tools. Like in *The Name of the Rose*[12] when Umberto Eco has the character based on William of Ockham say that we should recognize it's just a tool to get from one place to another and now we can get rid of it and we can find another tool. Theories are tools. They're supposed to have internal consistency and coherence. They make sense. They don't contradict themselves, but they're also supposed to have external correspondence. So, if you have the theory that the sun is really a chariot being pulled by a horse across the sky, maybe it helps a couple of thousand years ago. It gives you an idea why a ball of fire goes across the sky. But now we have more information that says that's not accurate. There's not a horse and a fire. And so every theory is not always good for everything – there is witchcraft and superstition. Science is good. But, in the area of psychology, a lot is perspective. Once when I was at another conference somebody came up to me and they said, "Are you Solution or are you Narrative?" You know, it was like asking are you Protestant or Catholic, are you Sunni or Shiite? Are you reformed, conservative or orthodox Jewish, which group are you? And if you're not in the right group, you're going to be in trouble. And I said, "Well, I'm just trying to help people and I use whatever I think could be helpful. You know, sometimes Solution is really good, but sometimes Narrative is really good, too."[13]

FLAVIO: You don't want to take a side.

MICHAEL: I don't want to pick a side – or better, I want to pick the side that helps and I want to avoid what hurts. So, I don't want to make people feel worse, or I think I helped them but now they feel that only I can help them, so they don't feel smarter or better. But I also know a lot and there are times I've said to somebody, "I don't understand why you would do that" or "That doesn't make sense to me." Like when I was talking about the young woman who was throwing up. I said, "You could do that, but I can tell you because I've known a lot of people, it gets worse and if you do that you'll get sick. You don't want to get sick, do you?" But this whole idea of one approach is very difficult.

FLAVIO: Sometimes I think that it's – it's simply math! I mean, there are hundreds of approaches – I've even heard that are more than one thousand. How can it be possible to think that there is *one* better than another? That CBT, or DBT, or ACT, or even Strategic Therapy or Solution-Focused Therapy is the best for everything and everyone? It's wrong math. It's like saying that there is only one perfect style of martial art.

MICHAEL: Or only one way to cook, or to make music.

FLAVIO: The question should be: "Perfect *for what?*" or "For *whom?*" I tend to think that one approach is good for one person but could be not so for another one.

MICHAEL: A related subject is why therapists do what they do, why we become psychodynamic or cognitive-behavioral or strategic, or systemic, or whatever else. I think there are several reasons. One reason is: it fits our personality. "I like to change my mind. I like to see things differently. I like to tell jokes." So, part of it is our energy, our style, our way of paying attention.

FLAVIO: I agree, and you did good to quote it first. As you know, I'm the Director of a post-degree school for psychologists,[14] and when we ask the students why they choose the school, often it is "Because I like the mood" or "Because it's a nice place." Of course, they trust the model – but the "mood" part, what fits with their taste, with their personality, seems to be very important, more so than research and data.

MICHAEL: Yes. And part of it is whom our teachers were when we went to school. A very important part, because the teachers tell us what's good and bad and they make fun of the ones that aren't good. They say, "Oh, it's too superficial," or maybe "It's too intellectual." So they make us feel what's right and wrong. And, as you said, occasionally people will say, "I actually read the research and found out what the best thing was." So occasionally it's partly based on evidence or research. Some of it is based on what clients want, but they've been taught by the movies and society what is good. I know when I was learning brief therapy, I wrote a paper called "Therapist Resistances to Short-Term Therapy."[15] We would think, "Oh, well, depth therapy and psychoanalysis, that's really the good stuff. And all this other stuff is a band-aid, or it's superficial, or it's not the really good stuff." I was once talking with somebody I knew, I said I was interested in brief therapy and he said, "Oh, I used to do that also, but now I do real therapy."

FLAVIO: Probably we have to shift our mind from which is "the real therapy," "the real theory," "the right theory," to which is the *useful* one, in this moment, for this client.

MICHAEL: But for many people, "real therapy" means deeper, childhood, crying, mother, trouble, painful, slow – that's "real."

FLAVIO: And that just was an idea developed by Freud and then taken by other therapists. In a chapter by Richard Fisch,[16] Fisch said "Therapies used to be short before Freud." It's provocative, I think, but it's true in a way. It reminds me that "therapy," the idea of therapy as a long-term treatment, is an idea, it's just an idea. And this reminds me about Jay Haley, who said that you need to be taught to do a long-term therapy – otherwise it is natural to do brief therapies.[17]

MICHAEL: Five hundred years ago, if I had a problem, I would go and talk to the shaman or the medicine man or woman or the guru or the chief or the village wise person. I would not expect that I'm going to go Tuesday at 10:00 for 50 minutes once a week for the next two years. I'm going to go have a meeting and it may not be 50 minutes, it may be all day. I may have to prepare myself to receive the message. I may have to fast or wear special clothes or take a drug or purify myself in some way and I would go, I would have an experience. And at the end of the experience, I would have ideas and things I'm supposed to do. It's not necessarily that everything is all instantly better, but we developed a very different way of thinking about therapy. I recall Haley[18] saying that the most important decision in the history of therapy was to charge by the hour. People come every week, week after week. They are taught to expect to go gradually and slowly. For some problems, it does take a long time. I'm not against therapy taking as long as it needs. I'm against therapy taking longer than it needs to take and I'm against telling people it has to be a long time. But if somebody has a bad problem and they have had it for many years, they may not in one hour be able to say, "Okay, I'm going to stop doing that, or I'm going to change the way I do that." At the Brief Therapy Conference I heard Robert Dilts give a very nice demonstration about helping people change self-limiting beliefs.[19] And he said, "You know, often times what we believe controls what we allow ourselves to think about, what to do." And he talked about it in therapy. We look for the fulcrum. The fulcrum is the balance point or the turning point. For some people that's their belief. Maybe it's a certain behavior, but if they change that, other things will change. So, you try to find the one thing, sometimes it's a belief.

FLAVIO: You talked about the "pivot chord."

MICHAEL: A pivot chord is like a fulcrum. The term *pivot chord* came from Bob Rosenbaum,[20] and a pivot chord is how you shift from one key to another in music. In therapy, it can be reframing or re-education, when a person sees things differently. Another related idea is sometimes we try to get the person to make a big dramatic shift; but other times, maybe just a small little change. Erickson said, "If you want people to make a big change, ask for a small change." Ericksonians[21] called this *progression*: do it just a little bit different, then a little bit more different, building incrementally on a small change. So, in one of the videotapes I show at conferences,[22] the woman finally says "No" to her father – he's very manipulative and controlling. Well, when she said "No" to her father, she also thinks, "Oh, I can say 'No' to my husband and I can say 'No' to my boss. I can say 'No' to my children. I can say 'No' to my family. I'm empowered." She got it with one experience with one person and then she generalized it. So sometimes it's very helpful to find something that the person can do to make a change that's not so big that it's impossible or it's too hard. A small change can lead to a big change.

FLAVIO: How do you find it? How do you find that pivot chord?

MICHAEL: "What would be one example of something you would like to do differently? When this problem is no longer a problem, what will be something we'll see you doing differently?"

FLAVIO: We, as therapists, we don't know if that is the fulcrum – that it's just the first step and if you make a little change other changes will follow. We don't know, for example, if a single session will be a single session until the end of the single session.

MICHAEL: There was a cartoon I saw in a magazine that I cut out and kept. A husband and wife are sitting in the kitchen and the wife is busy washing and cooking and preparing the food. And the husband is just sitting there reading the newspaper. I think they are leopards – leopards are the big cats with the spots on them, right? And the wife says, "I did not ask you to change your spots. I just asked you to wash the dishes." It's saying, "You don't have to be a completely different person. Just do this." It doesn't mean, "I'm not a man" or not whoever he thinks he is. In fact, you'll be a better leopard if you wash the dishes. So sometimes the person makes a little change, and that's all that's needed.

FLAVIO: Sometimes you're asked to do little things and sometimes a little thing can lead to a big change and sometimes it's a little thing that is connected to another little thing and another little thing and you can't know that before.

MICHAEL: So, another kind of pivot chord is *reframing*. Reframing, according to the people at MRI – Watzlawick, Weakland and Fisch[23] (1974) – means the same facts with a different meaning. To give an example: Michele Ritterman and I wrote a paper for the Erickson Newsletter a few years ago.[24] We were in a taxi with a driver and he was telling us about how he got divorced and he was very unhappy. His wife had left him and he'd been thinking about it for a long time. What kind of a terrible person would do that to him? We were riding in the taxi so I made it about him and told a joke about a taxi driver. I said:

> "You know the one about the taxi driver? He was driving his taxi and a policeman came up behind him and the cop pulled him over" (the taxi driver in the car with us looked around behind him to see what was going on) and the policeman, said, "I'm going to give you a ticket," and the cab driver said, "Oh, please don't give me a ticket. Please don't give me a ticket, please, please." And the policeman said, "Well, if you tell me a really good story, I won't give you a ticket." And the taxi driver said, "My wife ran away with a cop and when I saw you, I thought you were going to be bringing her back. I got scared!" And our driver laughed because what I said had reframed it: "Your wife being gone is not abandonment. Your wife being gone is escape. You no longer have to be with her as she's so bad she would do that to you." So we reframed the same fact that the wife left, but now he's rid of her, instead of he misses her. Now, did that solve all his problems? Probably not, but it gave him a different way of thinking about the situation: "He's right, I don't want to be around her. She was terrible to me. How could she do that?" And then he laughed, and he said, "I'm going to remember that!"

So that was a pivot chord. That was a moment when we looked at things differently. Here's another example of a pivot chord. In one of his books, Harry Stack Sullivan[25] talks about his doing an intake interview with a woman and she says, "You know, I'm kind of depressed. I'm smart, but I spend all my day being a housewife and I don't find it fulfilling. I'm bored." He listens to her and then he says, "The fact that you're bored and you're a little depressed is very good." She says, "It's good?" He says, "Yeah, it tells me that you have a lot of energy and intelligence that we have to find a better way to use. You're bored because you're smart and you want to do other things." So that's a pivot chord, where you pivot from it being a problem to seeing there is a strength inside the problem and we're going to use your strength. So that's a kind of a reframe again or a pivot chord. It leads to utilization. I think it's the therapist's job to help the client see herself or himself in a way that gives the client hope and a sense of "I could do something." For example, if somebody is obsessive, they notice little details all the time, I can say, "You know, it's very good you notice little details because that means you'll be able to follow instructions very carefully." Or somebody who's very emotional, instead of saying they're hysterical or histrionic, we could say: "You're very sensitive and in touch with your feelings. So, you will know what feels good and doesn't feel good. You can use this." Or if somebody is somewhat dependent, since "You're very good at noticing who in the situation could help you, who has resources and abilities that might help you, you'll be able to find a way to get them to help you."

FLAVIO: And often that is all we need, isn't it? "To solve the problem" is another mindset matter. If we think in the medical model mindset, we're tempted to say that we, as therapists, solve problems like medical doctors cure illnesses. You expect that the doctor will cure you and will follow you until the illness is totally gone. But if you are a psychotherapist, is it the same? What do we have to do to "solve" a problem? If we have this mindset we probably are damned to fail a lot of time. I've read that most therapies don't end with the therapist saying "The End": most of the time clients stop therapy when *they* think that that's it, they don't need other sessions.[26]

These are important questions: What is our purpose? Our goal? When is a therapy considered successful? And, decided by whom? Because probably it depends on the context. If we are doing a randomized clinical trial, to check the efficacy of a therapy, probably "success" corresponds to "the client attends until his/her symptoms are totally gone," otherwise it is a "drop-out" or a "failure." But I think that in private practice this often is not what happens. If you talk with those clients, those who interrupted the therapy before the therapist thought "The End," they will often say, "Oh, you know, I'm good now. Yes, I ended therapy before my therapist told me to do so, but it was good for me, and I'm good now." They could even say, "Yes, occasionally I have some symptoms, but my life is good, my relationships are good, my work is good, I feel good." So, was that an unsuccessful therapy? But, again, it's a mindset issue and it's important. Because we could say, "It doesn't matter what the client says. If the tests say that he still has some symptoms, then the therapy was unsuccessful," and this could drive future ideas about what psychotherapy is, what works, what mental illness is, what insurance should pay for and so go on.

MICHAEL: Yes, mindset can easily become ideology.

FLAVIO: Where are we?

MICHAEL: On Highway 1, in the county of Santa Barbara. We're not yet in the city of Santa Barbara. We're getting there. Santa Barbara County has a lot of agriculture and a lot of wineries. This is Guadalupe. Let's see – it says Highway One South. There are a couple of good ways we can go to get there.

FLAVIO: Hey, that's like a metaphor for what we've been talking about – different ways to get there, which detours to avoid!

MICHAEL: You think? [*laughs*]

FLAVIO: So, we said a lot; is there something else that you want to say about mindset?

MICHAEL: Be flexible. You don't want your mindset to be so set that it can't change. It's mindset, not mind-set-in-concrete.

FLAVIO: Maybe more than mindset, we have to talk about mind-*setting*.

MICHAEL: Yeah, that's a good way to look at it, as a verb, "mind setting." The basic mindset in brief therapy is: *Change is possible now or soon.* "You have an ability that I can help you recognize. Once you know what your goal is, you will be able to use your abilities. We can talk about how you're going to achieve your goal."

It's good to *pay attention to what you pay attention to.* How we make sense of our worlds – the stories we tell ourselves and each other – does much to determine what we experience, our actions and our destinies. Some stories are better than others because they are more enlivening and encouraging, helping people to get more of what they want. They carry wisdom and hope. They open people's hearts and touch their feelings. They speak to the person's truth or dream. They tap into our strengths and resources. They invigorate us, making us feel more alive and more deeply human. How we look influences what we see, and what we see influences what we do, 'round and around. What you focus on tends to grow, so be mindful of your mindset, your language and what you choose to emphasize.[27]

Techniques follow from your mindset. We have to do something with people. We can't just say, "Hi, how are you? Nice to see you." We have methods, strategies, approaches, techniques, procedures and processes – but they may not be important for exactly the reason we think they're important. What they tend to do, which is very important, is they give the client a focus, what they want to achieve, and they help the client and therapist to see what the client's resources or abilities are. That's what I've been calling the *Context of Competence*, where you help the client to bring resources and goals together via the therapeutic alliance.

To my mind, therapy takes place where Alliance/Goals/Resources overlap. If you identify Goals (or Problems) and have an Alliance but don't access Resources, nothing happens. If you have an Alliance and Resources but don't identify Goals (or Problems), there's nothing to do, no purpose. If the client could match up their Goals and Resources on their own, bringing to bear competencies to deal with problems, they wouldn't need the therapist. All three are often needed: the *Context of Competence* is where Goals and Resources come together through the Alliance. Effective therapy, one session or otherwise, involves all three.

Maybe next time we can talk more about techniques and the logics they serve.

Box 8. Context of Competence

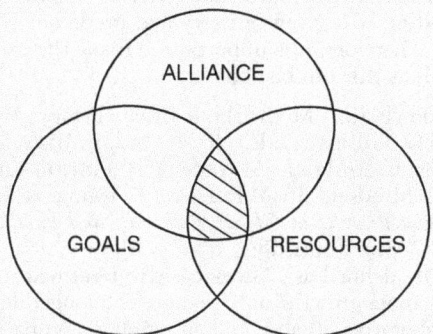

Figure 3.1 Context of Competence. (From M.F. Hoyt, 2014. "Psychology and My Gallbladder: An Insider's Account of a Single Session Therapy." In M.F. Hoyt & M. Talmon (Eds.), *Capturing the Moment: Single-Session Therapy and Walk-In Services* (pp. 53–72). Crown House Publishing. © M.F. Hoyt, 2014. Used with permission.

Box 9. Chapter 3 Summary: Mindset in Brief Therapy

The term *mindset* refers to a set of beliefs that influence how one thinks, feels, and behaves in any given situation. Through their dialogue, the authors explore how different mindsets can promote or impede efficient intervention and influence the length of therapy. Clinical examples are provided. The utility of conceiving a Context of Competence, in which Goals/Resources/Alliance intersect, is also discussed.

Reflection Question: What beliefs or expectations do you bring to a therapy session?

Notes

1 Hence, we believe that *mindset* is what John Weakland (1988, pp. 101–102, emphases in original) was referring to when he wrote about the "myths" that guide brief therapy:

> We do not live by realities, but by *interpretations* of observed events or situations. Even our observations – since we can never attend to everything fully and

equally – depend on preconceptions of what is most significant. […] Any such explanatory schema also proposes how the matter in question *should* be understood and responded to, and this is a directive outlining proper thought and action. Thus, in a fundamental sense myths are like maps; they shape and order our understanding of a given territory and guide our steps in traversing it, or avoiding it … Therefore, it is important to make the implicit content of myths explicit, as well as this can be done.

See J.H. Weakland (1988). "Myths about Brief Therapy, Myths of Brief Therapy." In J.K. Zeig & S.G. Gilligan (Eds.), *Brief Therapy: Myths, Methods, and Metaphors* (pp. 100–107). Brunner/Mazel. Also see: F. Cannistrà (2021). "The Vital Role of the Therapist's Mindset." In M.F. Hoyt, J. Young, & P. Rycroft (Eds.), *Single Session Thinking and Practice in Global, Cultural, and Familial Contexts: Expanding Applications* (pp. 77–88). Routledge.

2 *Brief therapy* can be defined as "Time-sensitive treatment to relieve psychological distress and/or promote growth" or (if you prefer a longer definition) as "The development of a collaborative alliance and an emphasis on patient/client strengths in the service of an efficient attainment of co-created goals" (M.F. Hoyt, 2009, *Brief Psychotherapies: Principles & Practices*. Zeig, Tucker, & Theisen).

3 M.F. Hoyt (2004). *The Present is a Gift: Mo' Better Stories from the World of Brief Therapy*. iUniverse.

4 See https://www.telegraph.co.uk/news/worldnews/europe/austria/1517214/Freuds-last-patient-recalls-meeting-that-saved-my-life.html.

5 Milton Erickson (quoted in Zeig, 1980, p. 148): "It is the patient who does the therapy. The therapist only furnishes the climate, the weather. That's all. The patient has to do all the work." See J.K. Zeig (1980). *A Teaching Seminar with Milton H. Erickson, M.D.* Brunner/Mazel. Also see pp. 14–15 and Chapter 6, this volume.

6 M.F. Hoyt (2017). "A Golfer's Guide to Brief Therapy (with Footnotes for Baseball Fans)." In *Brief Therapy and Beyond: Stories, Language, Love, Hope, and Time* (pp. 33–43). Routledge.

7 Michael later adds: When I was an intern at the University of Wisconsin, one of my supervisors had a needlepoint sign in his office that said "Bacon can be cured. People grow and change."

8 "The audacity of hope! In the end, that is God's greatest gift to us, the bedrock of this nation. A belief in things not seen. A belief that there are better days ahead." Barack Obama, Keynote Address, 2004 Democratic National Convention. Quoted in B. Obama & B. Springsteen (2021). *Renegades: Born in the USA* (p. v). Crown.

9 See M. White (1995). *Re-Authoring Lives: Interviews and Essays*. Dulwich Centre Publications; and M. White & D. Epston (1990). *Narrative Means to Therapeutic Ends*. Norton. Also see Hoyt (2017, op cit., pp. 104–109).

10 See M. Talmon & M.F. Hoyt (2014). "Moments Are Forever: SST and Walk-In Services Now and in the Future." In M.F. Hoyt & M. Talmon (Eds.) (2014), *Capturing the Moment: Single Session Therapy and Walk-In Services* (pp. 463–485). Crown House Publishing.

11 See Watzlawick (in Hoyt, 2001, p. 145). M.F. Hoyt (2001). "Constructing Therapeutic Realities: A Conversation with Paul Watzlawick." In M.F. Hoyt (Ed.), *Interviews with Brief Therapy Experts* (pp. 144–157). Brunner-Routledge.

12 U. Eco (1983). *The Name of the Rose*. Harcourt (published in Italian in 1980 as *Il Nome della Rosa*).

13 See M.F. Hoyt (2000). "Unmuddying the Waters: A 'Common Ground' Conference." In *Some Stories Are Better than Others* (pp. 195–200). Brunner/Mazel [work originally published 1997]. Also see: M.F. Hoyt (2019). "Strategic Therapies: Roots and Branches." *Journal of Systemic Therapies*, 38(1), 30–43.

14 The Italian Center for Single Session Therapy (in Rome). Visit www.singlesessiontherapies.com.
15 M.F. Hoyt (1985). "Therapist Resistances to Short-Term Dynamic Psychotherapy." *Journal of American Academy of Psychoanalysis, 13*(1), 93–112.
16 R. Fisch (1994). "Basic Elements in the Brief Therapies." In M.F. Hoyt (Ed.), *Constructive Therapies* (pp. 126–139). Guilford Press.
17 J. Haley (1990). "Why Not Long-Term Therapy?" In J.K. Zeig & S.G. Gilligan (Eds.), *Brief Therapy: Myths, Methods, and Metaphors* (pp. 3–17). Brunner/Mazel.
18 Haley (1990, pp. 14–15): "Historians will someday reveal who thought of this idea. The ideology and practice of therapy was largely determined when therapists chose to sit with a client and be paid for durations of time rather than by results." J. Haley (1990). "Why Not Long-Term Therapy?" op. cit.
19 R. Dilts. "Transforming Belief Barriers." Presentation at Brief Therapy Conference sponsored by Milton H. Erickson Foundation, Burlingame, CA, December 8, 2018.
20 R. Rosenbaum, M.F. Hoyt, & M. Talmon (1990). "The Challenge of Single-Session Therapies: Creating Pivotal Moments." In R.A. Wells & V.J. Giannetti (Eds.), *Handbook of the Brief Psychotherapies* (pp. 165–189). Plenum. Reprinted in M.F. Hoyt (1995). *Brief Therapy and Managed Care* (pp. 105–139). Jossey-Bass.
21 See D. Short, B.A. Erickson, & R.E. Klein (2005). *Hope and Resiliency: Understanding the Psychotherapeutic Strategies of Milton H. Erickson, M.D.* Crown House Publishing.
22 See M.F. Hoyt (2017). "A Single-Session Therapy Retold: Evolving and Restoried Understandings." In M.F. Hoyt, *Brief Therapy and Beyond* (pp. 134–152). Routledge.
23 "To reframe, then, means to change the conceptual and/or emotional setting or viewpoint in relation to which a situation is experienced and to place it in another frame which fits the 'facts' of the same concrete situation equally well or even better, and thereby changes its entire meaning." P. Watzlawick, J.H. Weakland, & R. Fisch (1974). *Change: Principles of Problem Formation and Problem Resolution.* Norton. See p. 95.
24 M.F. Hoyt & M. Ritterman (2012). "Brief Therapy in a Taxi." *The Milton H. Erickson Foundation Newsletter, 32*(2), 7.
25 H.S. Sullivan (1954). *The Psychiatric Interview.* Norton.
26 See pp. 9–10, M.F. Hoyt et al. (2018). "Introduction: Single-Session/One-at-a-Time Walk-In Therapy." In M.F. Hoyt, M. Bobele, A. Slive, J. Young, & M. Talmon (Eds.), *Single-Session Therapy by Walk-In Or Appointment* (pp. 3–24). Routledge. Also see M.F. Hoyt (2000). "The Last Session in Brief Therapy: How and Why to Say 'When.'" In M.F. Hoyt, *Some Stories Are Better Than Others* (pp. 237–261). Brunner/Mazel; and M.F. Hoyt & R. Rosenbaum (2018). "Some Ways to End an SST." In M.F. Hoyt, M. Bobele, A. Slive, J. Young, & M. Talmon. (Eds.), *Single-Session Therapy by Walk-In Or Appointment* (pp. 318–323). Routledge.
27 From p. 230, M.F. Hoyt (2017). *Brief Therapy and Beyond: Stories, Language, Love, Hope, and Time.* Routledge.

Chapter 4

Techniques and Logics in Brief Therapy

MICHAEL: So, what about technique, Flavio?

FLAVIO: I want to discuss the differences between techniques and logics.

MICHAEL: So the first definition: what is a *technique*? I think *technique* is a specific process. The Miracle Question could be a technique, or teaching someone a relaxation method could be a technique. Technique is something a technician could do. It's a specific procedure.

FLAVIO: I don't want to talk only about specific techniques but about the role of intervention. Techniques are important because otherwise you could simply say to a client "Hello" or talk about the weather.

MICHAEL: Techniques give the client something to focus on, an activity to do that involves them so that they feel they are participating and they are making a difference. They have some involvement. Techniques offer situations in which clients can be competent, they can do something.

Of course, it's not just the technique, but it's how skillfully the therapist – and the client – do the technique. A person saying, "Hey, what do you want?" is different from someone saying, "Suppose tonight, while you're sleeping, a miracle happens" – and they see the client look curious – "and when you wake up smiling, you begin to see things differently" – and the client's eyes brighten – "and what will be the first things you will see that says, 'Things are better?'" So how you deliver the technique is very important. The skillful communication of the technique is probably more important than the actual technique. The technique is not just the words, it's the relationship. It's how you deliver it. Do you deliver it in a way that captures the ear of the client, gets them to pay attention?

FLAVIO: Yes, and technique is not just the formal homework I give at the end of the session. "Technique" is also a category into which you can put a lot of interventions. Or, better, "interventions" is a category in which "technique" is just only one element. I mean that we can't reduce the session to the homework we give at the end of the session, or to the paradoxical sentence we maybe used at a precise point in the session, or to the role-playing we created during the session. Communication, tone of voice, the way we decide to relate with that particular client in that particular

DOI: 10.4324/9781003307709-5

moment – they all are "interventions" we do and that are important from a "technique" point of view of the therapy.

MICHAEL: There are lots of different kinds of techniques – like questioning and scaling, role-playing, using imagery, reframing, utilization, prescribing a symptom or an ordeal, telling a relevant joke, even yelling "Stop!"

FLAVIO: And I'm also thinking about Wampold's work again, and other similar ideas, which say that an important factor is how much the client believes in the model, in the technique. You must give them a rationale to believe in.[1] Often it's not the technique, it's the explanation of the technique: if the explanation makes sense and the client believes it. I don't completely agree with this – it seems to me that some techniques do what they do because of their particular structure, not just because they are delivered well or the client accepts them. From an interactional view it seems to me hard to accept that some of those techniques work "just because the client feels that he or she is doing *something.*" We know, from the systemic perspective, that if you change something in one element of the system than you change the system and the other elements. And it seems to me that this is what some techniques do. So... I don't know, just a reflection. Maybe I'll better understand this in the future.

MICHAEL: I agree. The content can be very important, like getting someone to see things differently, or to access and better use their abilities.

FLAVIO: But Wampold quotes some studies, called *dismantling studies*, in which they took away the main technique from a therapy – like gradual exposure to a phobic object – and the therapy works anyway, even without that basic technique. And I also can say for sure that the same technique usually doesn't work if you simply say, "Ok, do this, see you in two weeks, bye." It definitely is more likely to work if you present it with suggestive communication, with evocative language and so go on.

One of my favorite techniques, for example, is the *snap technique.* I don't want to startle you, so let's just say that the core of the technique is to snap your fingers and say "Michael! Come back here!" It is a very powerful technique for people who think too much – you know, mental ruminations, pathological doubting, that kind of thing. But I can't say, "OK, dear patient, in the next days, when you start doubting too much, snap your fingers, say your name and say 'Come back here.' That's it. See you in a couple of weeks. And here's my bill." I tried, and it doesn't work. I have to give a very complicated rationale and... no, it's not "complicated," but it must be persuasive, the client must agree with it. In fact I tend to ask him or her many feedback questions during my explanation: "Do you agree? Does it make sense for you?" etc. So, how you communicate a technique is very, very important.

MICHAEL: My colleague Monte Bobele likes to quote his mentor Harry Goolishian, who advised, "A good intervention is like a kitchen match – it only works once."[2] Many times people do something and it works, so they start to do it with all of their clients and it doesn't work as well because now it doesn't fit the context. The first time, it was fresh and original. It was exciting. It was interesting to that client. But if a technique becomes automatic or rote, it is no longer really an effective technique.

I once had a client sitting in my office. We had been working very hard on her problems with relationships and trusting people and she had met a guy. She liked him. She went out on a date with him and she had a good time, and then a couple of days later when she talked to him, she found out that he already had a girlfriend and he was cheating on her. She was very disappointed. When she told me I stood up and I kicked the wall in my office. I said, "Damn it!" She laughed and it was clear that I was disappointed for her. I actually kicked the wall. Not too hard, but hard enough – it made a noise. So, is that the technique: kick a wall when the patient gives you bad news? No. It was showing solidarity with the patient by showing that I was also disappointed. I had never before and have never since kicked the wall with anybody. I could have said sympathetically, "Oh, that's disappointing." Or I could've said, "That guy was a jerk." My kick-the-wall-damn-it response was spontaneous and genuine, which made it more authentic and significant (and probably, more memorable). They're all different things, but the underlying idea of the logic was to show support, and the technique was how to do it.

Box 10. Logic: The Reason That Underlies a Particular Behavior and That Justifies It

The term *logic* can include meanings like reason, purpose, intention, desired result/effect, goal, etc. The basic idea is that when a therapist does (or assigns) a specific intervention or uses a specific tactic, it is because he or she means to achieve a specific effect. The therapist has the idea that the intervention will act in a specific way, hoping that following a logic will bring the desired result. See Chapter 8 in which the authors describe nine different logics that guide different interventions in brief therapies.

So, I think techniques have to be guided by what you are trying to accomplish. What is your *logic* or your purpose or objective? You could ask the Miracle Question, or you could ask "What are your best hopes for what you want to get from this meeting?" or "When you leave, what will tell you it was worth coming to see me and spending time and money today?" They're all different techniques, but they're all serving the logic of setting a goal or a purpose or a direction. Or you could use humor, maybe even tell a carefully selected joke – the logic could be to build the relationship or to suggest a different awareness (construction/interpretation) of what's going on, or to block something – different purposes can be served by the same technique. So, I think sometimes people say, "I have to learn 100 techniques or 700 techniques." There are many techniques. There are books on family therapy techniques, cognitive-behavioral therapy techniques, how to do joining maneuvers, how to do paradoxes and how to do confrontations, and it's good to have skills – but the techniques are for a purpose, so you have to know your purpose.

FLAVIO: I totally agree. This fits with the idea of the "9 Logics" and with the work we're doing about that.[3] Many common factors therapists say that hope is an important common factor, that the client hopes that the therapy will work. So are you also saying that probably the technique is a way to say "You're doing something and this will help you"?

MICHAEL: Yes, but I'm saying even more. Whatever technique we're doing, if I'm the client and I'm doing the technique with Flavio, I'm thinking "Now we're doing the therapy that he knows will help me." So, it's not just the technique. It's giving me hope because I'm participating with "The Expert." The Doctor has a treatment for me and we're doing it so I'm going to get better. The treatment could be waving his hand back and forth. It could be writing in my journal. It could be burning a letter, it could be thinking about a time I was happy, it could be learning a new way to talk with my partner, but whatever it is it gives me encouragement just because it's a technique that the doctor has prescribed or the doctor has directed. That's Jerome Frank in *Persuasion and Healing*[4] talking about rituals and restoring morale.

FLAVIO: What do you think about those techniques that set standards? For example, you can use exposure techniques, or you can use paradoxical intention for anxiety or to avoid panic attacks. What do you think about it? You're saying that techniques are important and that part of their usefulness is that you are putting the client in the mode of doing something – but there are also some techniques that are used by all different types of therapists as a sort of standard: "If you have this problem, then I'll use this technique." What do you think about it?

MICHAEL: Many roads lead to Rome. Learning to face one's fears is useful, whether we call it exposure and response prevention, desensitization, insight, opposite action, blocked unsuccessful attempted solutions, or whatever. This is where theory comes in. If the theory guides the therapist to the technique then the therapist will believe in the technique, and when the therapist believes in the technique, the client will believe in the technique because the therapist is confident. The therapist thinks, "This is a really good technique that I'm giving you" and the client thinks, "This is a really good technique that she's giving me."

FLAVIO: Oh, this is brilliant, Michael! With just a few words you also explained why different problems can be solved by different techniques or protocols. And, furthermore, it opens an interesting perspective: often ourselves as therapists tend to believe that a technique is the standard, it is what works more than everything. … Actually, that's what is taught mostly.

MICHAEL: There was an article I read some years ago[5] that said when a new medicine comes out and the doctors believe in it the patients get better and then after a few years when they begin to use it a lot, it doesn't always work as well. The patients stop getting better. Part of it is the actual medicine, and part of it is the way I deliver it to you: "I just read the latest research article and this medicine is going to cure you. I'm an expert and of all the things in the world, this is what is best for you." So, I think the technique is important – especially if you believe it! You could do therapy with a computer and it will say, "Think of a scary situation. We'll teach you how to relax. Think of a scary situation. Breathe slowly, relax your muscles. Think about…" You might say, "Well, but there's no relationship." But the client does have a relationship, they have it with the computer. The computer is an expert. Their transference is not to a person, it's to the cyber-authority. The machine is an expert, and the machine is telling me what to do. And computers are seen as having searched all the databases for what is best. So I think part of it is getting the client to believe in the technique, that this will help you. But then I do think certain techniques do work better than others. If I'm trying to teach somebody to relax, there may be different ways – like progressive muscle relaxation, certain ways of breathing, distraction, using positive imagery to think of a relaxing situation. But I think the technique always comes from the therapist. My colleague Terry Soo-Hoo[6] likes to say that the therapist is the therapy. I generally agree – the therapy comes through the therapist – but for most of us it's not just enough to be nice or loving or kind. I have heard reports about certain therapists and certain other people, if you were with them, you would feel better just by being in the room with them. You would feel better. Some of them are gurus and healers. Just to be with them, you're more honest or you're healthier or they see you with love in their eyes and you feel like a worthwhile person. I heard Arnold Lazarus, the cognitive-behavioral therapist, say that the therapeutic alliance is the soil in which techniques may grow, but if there is no good alliance, no good soil, the techniques will fall on hard ground and they will not blossom and they will not be helpful.

FLAVIO: So, we need to ask both *Why?* and *How?* The *Why?* is to consider the purpose of a technique, what is our intention, what are we trying to accomplish? And the *How?* is the way the therapist works with dialogue, questions, the relationship, the client's resources, etc., to make the difference. It seems that "formal techniques" are a concentrate of knowledge, like complexity reducers: they are important, but they don't do all the job.

MICHAEL: But even if the "common factors" research says that "therapist techniques" only account for a percentage of outcome variance, I think that what we do as therapists is important. We don't "cure" or "fix" people, but the therapist's techniques can build alliance and help to bring out the client's contributions.

FLAVIO: If techniques count just for a part, and the alliance or therapist-client relationship makes a bigger difference, we really need to re-think psychotherapy.

MICHAEL: It's important to do what works and not blame the client if/when something isn't successful.

FLAVIO: Just a last question. You use different kind of approaches and that means different kind of techniques. Do you have some preferred approaches for particular clients? Like: "With these kinds of clients I prefer Strategic Therapy. With those others I think it's better to use Solution-Focused Brief Therapy," etc. How do you choose which approach to use? Do you have some particular techniques that are personal favorites?

MICHAEL: That's a big question! Let me first start with some generalities. In *Problem-Solving Therapy*, Haley said "If therapy is to end properly, it must begin properly – by negotiating a solvable problem and discovering the social situation that makes the problem necessary."[7] The basic action-oriented MRI question is thus: "*Who* is doing *what* that presents a problem to *whom*, and *how does such a behavior constitute a problem?*" So, #1: I like to *ask the client what they are looking for* and, if they have been in therapy previously, *what was helpful* – their answers can give some ideas of what's likely to be useful (and what wasn't useful).[8]

FLAVIO: I totally agree! This is to me the essence of a good single-session therapy: help the clients to find what is useful for them and how they can use it again. It's similar to a solution-focused mindset, but possibly different in the methods by which you achieve it – I believe that the clients are the experts of their lives, but I don't exclude the therapist from the equation, if he/she can suggest some ways to be helpful. Of course, you must follow ethical principles, but when you're doing that then there are moments in which you can be briefer simply by suggesting things like "Hey, you did it before. Can we arrange a way to do it again?" I think we discussed that before.

MICHAEL: Yes. #2: *explanation leads to recognition, but experience leads to change* – meaning, it's good to help the client have a new experience, not just to become aware of what is wrong – so it's good to get him/her/them to practice doing something differently.

FLAVIO: Yes! And here's the point I mentioned before. It's ethical to help the client to find for themselves what can be helpful for them. But is it ethical if you have an idea of what that can be and you don't suggest that idea because "the client must reach that idea by themselves"? I think that labeling and psychological colonization are bad things we need to avoid, of course, and therapists sometimes are not aware about their communications or behaviors that can be sexist or racist.[9] So the therapist has to be careful to respect the client and help him/her in the best possible way. Paraphrasing Watzlawick,[10] it is helpful and probably is the best thing to help a person to learn to swim, but if she's drowning probably it's better to give her a lifebelt or even to dive into the water and bring her to shore.

MICHAEL: Here's a somewhat unusual example. I intermittently saw a fellow, let's call him "Richard." We met when his first marriage was ending; then later, when he was dating; and then later, when he had met a new woman and they were engaged and going to get married. I then didn't see him for quite a while, until one day he made an appointment. He had married and they were happy – but at the end of the session he mentioned that there was a woman he had met through work who was very attractive and she was flirting with him and he was tempted. He looked at me and said, "What do you think?" And I looked back and said, "Richard, are you out of your fucking mind?" He looked a bit startled, then laughed and said, "I didn't think you'd give a thumbs up." We shook hands, and that was our last session.

FLAVIO: Do you know what happened?

MICHAEL: So maybe three years later I was going to go to a movie. I got there early and went for a little walk. And I heard on the sidewalk behind me, "Hey, Michael!" I turned and it was Richard. We chatted. I said "I wondered whatever happened after our last session." Richard smiled. He took out his cellphone and showed me some pictures of his wife with their two young children. "I owe you a big 'Thank You,'" he said. "I remember what you said – when I needed it, you gave me the kick of approval."

FLAVIO: Wow!

MICHAEL: Yeah. "The kick of approval." I'm not saying you should swear and curse at clients, but Richard and I knew each other and we were "two guys" and I don't think it would have had much impact if I had said something benign but less impactful, like "I'm wondering why you're asking me this?" or "How would having an affair with that woman align with your intentions to have a happy marriage and family?" or even, "What are some other situations when you've used good judgment and resisted temptation?"

FLAVIO: That was an example of the logic "Direct Block of Actions."

MICHAEL: I think so. So continuing, #3: While I'm interested in second-order change, modifying problem-generating intrapsychic and interpersonal rules, with experience I have tended to *focus more on pragmatics, on what small, specific modifications might be made* with the hope that they may ripple out into larger life patterns.[11]

FLAVIO: Sorry – may I interrupt you again?

MICHAEL: Sure. Don't worry – go for it!

FLAVIO: A colleague of mine, Fabio Leonardi,[12] got me to reflect on something very interesting. To change behaviors influences *both* intrapsychic and interpersonal rules. The old saying that "You just cure the symptoms, but you don't address the unconscious dynamics" is wrong, because it implies that the symptoms, the "surface," is unrelated to the unconscious, the "depth." In that erroneous way, one could also say something like, "You just cure the unconscious dynamics. You don't address the symptom." Those are words I don't usually use – *unconscious, surface, depth* – they belong to a different vocabulary than mine. But if a critic were to say "You stay on the surface and don't address the depth" that would probably be what I'd say.

MICHAEL: That is an interesting point – "intrapsychic" and "interpersonal" are like sides of a coin.

So, on to #4: It's often good to *cultivate the client's motivation* – "If you don't change directions, you're going to wind up where you're heading" is a phrase that has encouraged lots of folks to make the effort to change; and

#5: It's important to *help facilitate the client using whatever happened in the office outside the office.* How can we help them to recall and apply the lessons of therapy when they really need them in the real world? "Termination" means "extracting the therapist from the successful equation",[13] essentially asking "You've been doing well with me, how will you continue to do well without me? Which of the helpful things you've been doing do you think you should continue to do? How can you do this?"

These are broad generalities, of course – one size doesn't fit all – and we can become better therapists by conscientiously paying attention to what works and what doesn't. When we learn a new technique, we often want to use it almost all the time – like a kid with a new toy.[14]

So... favorite techniques? In golf it's good to know where the hole is, so in therapy identifying the client's goals and hopes and motivating reasons: why it would be good to change, and asking what they've tried and how that went. Some typical questions might include: What's the problem, and for whom? Why have you called now (rather than last week, or waiting awhile longer)? When the problem isn't so bad, what are you doing differently then? In the middle of each session and the middle of a therapy, reframing and utilization can be very useful, as well as enactments/role-playing/practice, and checking to make sure you and the client are going in the direction the client wants to go.

Then there's checking on progress and planning possible next steps. Late in a session and in a therapy, termination becomes central, so it's important to help facilitate the client using whatever happened in the office outside the office. How can we help them to recall and apply the lessons of therapy when they really need them in the real world? Some useful guideline questions might include:

* Has this been helpful to you – and how so?
* Which of the helpful things that you've been doing do you think you should continue to do? –
* And how will you overcome obstacles that will come up?

* Who will be glad to hear about your progress?
* How will you remember to use the things we've been talking about, when you really need them?

As my colleague Bob Rosenbaum[15] once wrote, some people need to remember to remember, some need to remember to forget, some need to forget to remember, and some need to forget to forget!

FLAVIO: Do you have any favorite case stories?

MICHAEL: I've published a number of case studies and clinical vignettes that illustrate different techniques with individuals and couples.[16] Generally speaking, I have moved toward solution-focused/solution-oriented strengths and competence-based approaches. When I was at Kaiser, however, I was the designated OCD specialist in our clinic, and with those folks I found – even before knowing about Nardone's work on OCD[17] – that a strategic approach in which we deliberately blocked unsuccessful attempted solutions worked better than simply (or not so simply) trying to support the clients' solution efforts – which often involved avoidance. What we did may have looked to a CBT- or DBT-oriented therapist like "exposure and response prevention,"[18] but there were also strong elements of solution, narrative, Ericksonian and paradoxical approaches – all with a good dollop of humor. How you look influences what you see – a psychodynamicist observing a two-chair Gestalt therapy process might see "transference" being enacted; a redecision therapist (à la the Gouldings) might ask, "Who's been living in your head?"; a cognitively oriented therapist might describe the same clinical interaction in terms of "maladaptive self-schemas"; a narrative therapist might talk about "personification," "externalization" and "relative influence questioning"; an existentialist would talk about "choice" and "meaning-making"; a solution-oriented therapist might understand the second-chair persona as an "exception" to the problem; an Ericksonian might focus on the hypnotic suggestion of a new experience; and an MRI therapist might conceptualize the process as the disruption of a positive feedback loop and the evocation of second-order change.

FLAVIO: So: "How you look influences what you see –"

MICHAEL: "– and what you see influences what you do, 'round and around."

Box 11. Chapter 4 Summary: Techniques and Logics in Brief Therapy

Techniques have always been a central topic of various brief therapy discourses. The authors have an in-depth dialogue about their role, purpose, relevance, and uses. Both *why* and *how* a certain technique is delivered – the context, the therapist's skillfulness, and the client's receptiveness –

will influence its effectiveness. Specific interventions and the various intentions that guide them are explored, with clinical examples.

Reflection Question: Describe a technique you have used and how in different situations it could serve different purposes (e.g., to build alliance, establish a goal, block an unsuccessful attempted solution, identify a strength, etc.).

Notes

1 See B.E. Wampold & Z.E. Imel (2015). *The Great Psychotherapy Debate: The Evidence for What Makes Psychotherapy Work* (2nd ed.). Routledge. Also see J.D. Frank & J.B. Frank (1991). *Persuasion and Healing: A Comparative Study of Psychotherapy* (3rd ed.). Johns Hopkins University Press.
2 See p. 216 in M.F. Hoyt & M. Bobele (Eds.), *Creative Therapy in Challenging Situations: Unusual Interventions to Help Clients*. Routledge.
3 See F. Cannistrà (2019). "A Violent Life: Using Brief Therapy 'Logics' to Facilitate Change." In M.F. Hoyt & M. Bobele (Eds.), *Creative Therapy in Challenging Situations: Unusual Interventions to Help Clients* (pp. 47–57). Routledge. See also Chapter 8, this volume.
4 J.D. Frank & J.B. Frank (1991). *Persuasion and Healing: A Comparative Study of Psychotherapy* (3rd ed.). Johns Hopkins University Press.
5 J. Lehrer (2010, December 10). "The Truth Wears Off." *The New Yorker*, 52–57.
6 T. Soo-Hoo (2019). "Beyond Reason and Insight: The 180-Degree Turn in Therapeutic Interventions." In M.F. Hoyt & M. Bobele (Eds.), *Creative Therapy in Challenging Situations: Unusual Interventions to Help Clients* (pp. 193–208). Routledge.
7 See p. 9 in J. Haley (1977). *Problem-Solving Therapy: New Strategies for Effective Family Therapy*. Jossey-Bass.
8 Remember de Shazer's (quoted in Hoyt, 1996, p. 68) rules from solution-focused brief therapy:

> "(1)If it ain't broke, don't fix it; (2)Once you know what works, do more of it; and (3)If it doesn't work, don't do it again; do something different.

See M.F. Hoyt (1996). "Solution Building and Language Games: A Conversation with Steve de Shazer." In M.F. Hoyt (Ed.), *Constructive Therapies* (Vol. 2, pp. 60–85). Guilford Press.
9 See, for example, B.J. Mallinger & J.S. Lamberti (2010). "Psychiatrists' Attitudes toward and Awareness about Racial Disparities in Mental Health Care." *Psychiatric Services*, 61(2), 173–179; D.W. Sue & D. Sue (Eds.) (2007). *Counseling the Culturally Diverse* (5th ed.). Wiley; J. Owen, K.W. Tao, Z.E. Imel, B.E. Wampold, & & E. Rodolfa (2014). "Addressing Racial and Ethnic Microaggressions in Therapy." *Professional Psychology: Research and Practice*, 45(4), 283–290.
10 G. Nardone & P. Watzlawick (1993). *The Art of Change*. Jossey-Bass.
11 The Gouldings' *contract question* ("What are you willing to change today?") is often helpful. See M.M. Goulding & R.L. Goulding (1979). *Changing Lives through Redecision Therapy*. Brunner/Mazel. Also see Chapter 5 (pp. 92–100) this volume.
12 In 2019 Fabio published a very interesting book, unfortunately thus far only in Italian (*La Psicoterapia tra Miti e Realtà – Psychotherapy between Myths and Realities*), but he's also the author of several articles in English.

13 J.P. Gustafson (1986). *The Complex Secret of Brief Therapy.* Norton. Also see M.F. Hoyt (2017). "The Last Session in Brief Therapy: How and Why to Say 'When.'" In *Brief Therapy and Beyond* (pp. 153–176). Routledge; and M.F. Hoyt & R. Rosenbaum (2018). "Some Ways to End an SST." In M.F. Hoyt. M. Bobele, A. Slive, J. Young, & M. Talmon (Eds.), *Single-Session Therapy and Walk-in Services* (pp. 318–323). Routledge.

14 For more "helpful hints" see Hoyt (2017, *op cit.,* pp. 216–231).

15 R. Rosenbaum, M.F. Hoyt, & M. Talmon (1990). "The Challenge of Single-Session Therapies: Creating Pivotal Moments." In R.A. Wells & V.J. Gianneti (Eds.), *Handbook of the Brief Psychotherapies* (pp. 165–189). Plenum. Reprinted, with changes, in M.F. Hoyt, *Brief Therapy and Managed Care* (pp. 105–139). Jossey-Bass.

16 For some examples, see Hoyt (2017, *op. cit.*); Hoyt & Bobele (2019, *op. cit.);* and M.F. Hoyt (2015). "Solution-Focused Couple Therapy." In A.S. Gurman, J.L. Lebow, & D.K. Snyder (Eds.), *Clinical Handbook of Couple Therapy* (5th ed., pp. 300–332). Guilford Press.

17 For some recent examples of supporting research, see G. Pietrabissa, G.M. Manzoni, P. Gibson, D. Boardman, A. Gori, & G. Castelnuovo (2016). "Brief Strategic Therapy for Obsessive-Compulsive Disorder: A Clinical and Research Protocol of a One-Group Observational Study." *BMJ Open, 6*(3), e009118; G. Vitry, C. de Scorraille, & M.F. Hoyt (2021). "Redundant Attempted Solutions: 50 Years of Theory, Evolution, and New Supporting Data." *Australian and New Zealand Journal of Family Therapy, 42,* 174–187; and G. Vitry, C. de Scorraille, C. Portelli, & M.F. Hoyt (2021). "Redundant Attempted Solutions: Operative Diagnosis and Strategic Interventions to Disrupt More of the Same." *Journal of Systemic Therapies, 40*(4), 11–28.

18 See K. Rowa, M.M. Antony, & R.P. Swinson (2007). "Exposure and Response Prevention." In M.M. Antony, C. Purdon, & L.J. Summerfeldt (Eds.), *Psychological Treatment of Obsessive-Compulsive Disorder: Fundamentals and Beyond* (pp. 79–109). American Psychological Association.

Chapter 5

A Brief History of Brief Therapy, Some Personal Influences, and Thoughts about the Future

FLAVIO: I like your "brief history of brief therapy" in the *Brief Psychotherapies* book. It helped me to have a frame. So I think it could be useful to talk a little about history. How did therapy become brief?

MICHAEL: We usually think of psychotherapy as starting with Freud in the 1890s-1900 and then onward. As I wrote in *Brief Psychotherapies: Principles & Practices*,[1] Freud's early cases were brief – even single sessions, like Katarina and Mahler.

FLAVIO: Yes. And that other case report, the one about the woman who reported that when she was a child her mother had died and her father was being overprotective of the girl (probably because of his own grief) and Freud instructed her to tell her father to allow her to watch programs that showed romance?

MICHAEL: Right. Freud came right to the point.

FLAVIO: So then maybe the question really is: How did therapy become *long*?

MICHAEL: Psychoanalysis was just being developed and was being used as a research instrument, and they were discovering that if the therapist would remain a relatively passive "blank" screen, treatment took longer and longer and phenomena seemed to emerge like transference and the oedipal complex. Some early efforts to have the therapist be active were tried, most notably by Otto Rank and Sandor Ferenczi, but some of their methods were questionable (like having a patient sit on the therapist's lap), and the time for revisionism wasn't ripe because psychoanalysis was still struggling to establish itself. Even Freud (1937), in his last great paper, *Analysis Terminable and Interminable*, complained about relatively limited therapeutic benefits and called for the development of new methods based on psychodynamic principles.

FLAVIO: So why is psychoanalysis still a long-term therapy?

MICHAEL: Sometimes people's problems and their situations – their internal and external challenges and resources – are difficult, but a lot of what determines the length of therapy is some combination of theory, mindset, and an overly broad (read: dubious) mission – plus economics.

FLAVIO: Please continue telling about the history.

DOI: 10.4324/9781003307709-6

MICHAEL: A major influence toward briefer therapy was World War II. Until then, psychotherapy was mostly a long-term luxury for the well-to-do, but the war was on and "shell-shocked" (now called "PTSD") soldiers needed to be taken care of and, when possible, returned to the fighting – and so several things resulted in the United States: (1) psychologists and social workers became therapy providers and not just respective psych-testers and home-visitors; (2) group therapy became much more popular; and (3) the Veterans Administration (VA) medical system emerged and became a major treatment and training venue. More emphasis was put on "coping" and "ego functions," and efficiency and "reality factors" (like money and return to work) became more significant.

FLAVIO: It's amazing, isn't it? We say that things work in a specific way and that is the only possible way they can work in. And then there's something completely unexpected or out of our control – like the war – and that helps us to see things in a new light, and what was "impossible" is now necessary.

MICHAEL: In English we have the old saying, "Necessity is the mother of invention." You could also say, "Necessity is the mother of intervention"!

FLAVIO: Ha!

MICHAEL: So, back to the history. In 1946, Franz Alexander and Thomas French published their famous book, *Psychoanalytic Therapy: Theory and Application.*[2] They coined the phrase "corrective emotional experience" and advocated that therapists should modify their behavior (like being strict or indulgent) to fit individual patients. In the 1950s different workers were exploring ways to make psychodynamic therapy more focused and shorter-term. At the same time, Fritz Perls and his associates were developing Gestalt Therapy, Al Ellis was developing Rational-Emotive Therapy (the first systematic form of CBT), and Eric Berne was developing Transactional Analysis. There were lots of folks trying to make therapy more what we now sometimes call "time-sensitive," that is, more effective and efficient.

FLAVIO: I've also read somewhere that in the United States you had something like the National Mental Health Act – I'm not sure about the name. And also that the feminist movement was important for the development of briefer methods of psychotherapy, is that right?

MICHAEL: Back in the early 1970s there was parity legislation called the HMO Acts that said federally regulated health maintenance organizations (HMOs) had to offer the same level of care for mental or psychological conditions as they did for physical conditions. This may have helped encourage the development of more efficient approaches for long-term or chronic problems, including more use of intermittent therapy throughout the life cycle.[3] The feminist movement has made many contributions, including emphasizing the importance of self-determination and focusing on competence and strengths as well as questioning patriarchal assumptions about gender and power and what is "normal" and who decides.

There was also the "managed care" movement, which I discussed in *Brief Therapy and Managed Care*.[4] Steven Friedman and I wrote about some of the ethical dilemmas.[5] There have been various problems with managed care – I have sometimes called it "mangled care" – but in terms of brief therapy, a further emphasis was being put on efficient results and accountability. In 1988 the Milton H. Erickson Foundation held the first Brief Therapy Conference in San Francisco – my co-presenters Moshe Talmon and Bob Rosenbaum and I gave our first paper on Single Session Therapy (SST). There have been many Brief Therapy conferences since.

Box 12. Managed Care

Psychotherapy under managed care involves arrangements that regulate the utilization, site and costs of services; the nature and length of mental health treatment is determined partially by parties (insurers and reviewers) other than the clinician and patient/client. Brief (or short-term) therapy, which is the backbone of such arrangements, is defined not by a particular number of sessions but rather by the intention of helping patients make changes in thoughts, feelings, and actions in order to move forward or reach a particular goal as time-efficiently as possible.[6]

FLAVIO: Including the one in Burlingame, where we both were speakers.
MICHAEL: Indeed! Especially important for our interests, in the early 1950s Gregory Bateson, who was an anthropologist/philosopher, was studying communication. He got a research grant and sent Jay Haley and John Weakland to see what this fellow, Milton Erickson, was doing out in Arizona. This led to whole different ways of thinking about problems and solutions – cybernetics and interactional influence, looking at what was going on in the present that maintained a problem rather than assuming problems resided in the individual's past. Erickson also changed the emphasis from the unconscious as a place of conflicts and problems to a place of unappreciated capacities and potential solutions – which led to the idea of *utilization*. Haley eventually edited three volumes of *Conversations with Milton H. Erickson, M.D.* as well as his classic *Uncommon Therapy: The Psychiatric Techniques of Milton H. Erickson, M.D.*[7]

The Mental Research Institute (MRI) in Palo Alto, California, was founded in 1959 by Don Jackson, who had worked with Harry Stack Sullivan. Dick Fisch started to direct the Brief Therapy Center there; Haley and many other people were there – Paul Watzlawick, John Weakland, Cloé Madanes and Virginia Satir; others like R.D. Laing, Irvin Yalom and Salvador Minuchin came to visit. When I asked Jay, many years later, why they called it "Brief Therapy," he said it was mostly just to distinguish it from long-term (then mostly psychoanalytic) therapy. Steve de Shazer and Insoo Berg also studied at MRI – Steve (de Shazer, 1982) wrote *Patterns of Brief Family Therapy*, in which they were doing strategic therapy, assigning directives to counter problems, but then he got more focused on solution formation and developed SFBT. The first time I taught at MRI, on the wall in the seminar room facing me were photos of Jackson, Bateson, Erickson, Haley, Watzlawick, Weakland, Fisch, Satir and other "first-generation" luminaries – it was a bit overwhelming: I felt like my heroes and bibliography were watching me!

FLAVIO: I remember meeting you in that room!

MICHAEL: Yeah. We had previously exchanged some emails, but you came all the way from Rome to Palo Alto, California. You walked in and we both said *"Ciao!"*

FLAVIO: Right! How do you see Erickson's influence?

MICHAEL: I never personally met Erickson, but for many of us, Milton Erickson was like Zeus – realms of hypnotherapy, strategic therapy, brief therapy, and family therapy seem to have emerged from his forehead (in the Greek legend, creation also came from Zeus' thigh – which, in my poetic mind, maybe has to do with Erickson having polio and being in a wheelchair, so he learned to observe carefully and use language skillfully to get people to do things). Many books have been written about Erickson.

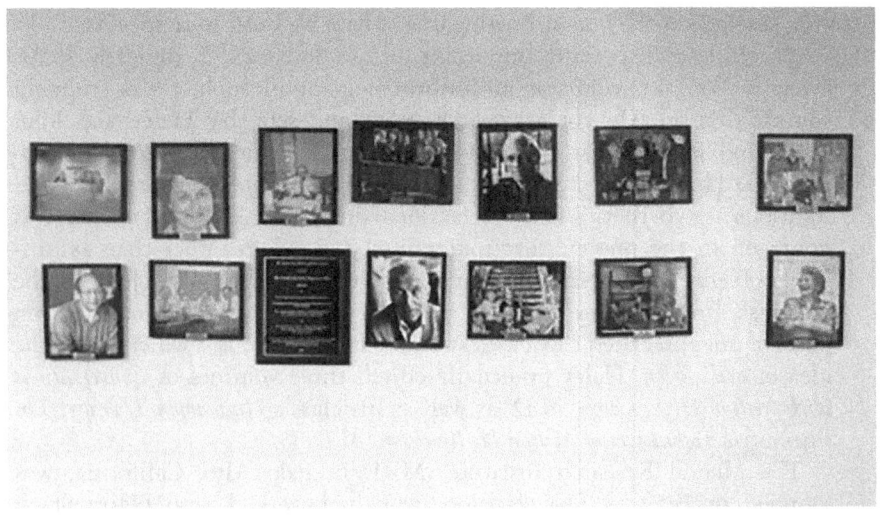

Figure 5.1 Wall at MRI. Pictures include Jay Haley, John Weakland, Milton Erickson and Gregory Bateson, Dick Fisch, Paul Watzlawick, and Virginia Satir. Photo kindly provided by Karin Schlanger (2020). ©Karin Schlanger. Used with permission.

Haley's *Uncommon Therapy* is probably the most famous and the best place to start; the ones called *Taproots* by Bill O'Hanlon and *Hope and Resiliency* by Dan Short and two of Erickson's daughters are for me the clearest in terms of identifying themes in Erikson's work, along with Rubin Battino and Thomas South's textbook-manual.[8] One of Erickson's best students was Michele Ritterman – her idea that symptoms are family and socially induced trance states is fascinating, and she wrote a book[9] that integrates the exterior-structural therapy viewpoint and the interior-hypnotherapy viewpoint.

Erickson was a giant with many contributions. I think his two most important legacies today are (1) *speak the client's language*, meaning enter into the client's worldview; and (2) the idea of *utilization*, to use whatever the client brings, the client's own abilities, to solve their problems. That's why I wanted to quote him several times and emphasize the shift toward the positive at the beginning of the SST paper we coauthored for the Italian journal (see Chapter 6). Erickson's ideas about using strategic directives and his work with hypnosis and non-trance communication as suggestion are also groundbreaking.

FLAVIO: Yeah, I agree. And how about John Weakland's role? I think he deserves more credit than is recognized.

MICHAEL: My understanding is that Weakland was hired by Bateson, along with Haley, to study Erickson – and, as Haley reported in *Conversations with Milton H. Erickson, M.D.*, they spent many weeks over several years visiting and learning from Erickson. The people who really knew John hold him in the highest regard; but in general Weakland is somewhat underappreciated, because he was not as dramatic as some of the others. I remember John commenting that his low-key style didn't get the big keynote speaker fees. John had started out as a chemical engineer, very scientific, and then had switched and was working on a combined sociology/anthropology PhD when he went to work with Bateson and then helped found the Brief Therapy Center at MRI. The two great books from MRI, *Change* (1974) and *The Tactics of Change* (1982), both have John Weakland as a coauthor. John was also a coauthor, with Bateson, Jackson and Haley, of the famous "double-bind" paper.

John was very smart and subtle. I think John's greatest contribution, among many, was clear-thinking and his emphasis on careful observation, on seeing what really was going on rather than on starting with an *a priori* theory or hypothesis and just looking for confirmation of what one wants to see.[10] It is significant that John and the early MRI group, along with Carl Rogers, were among the first to actually audiotape sessions so that they could repeatedly review them to learn what had made a difference. Their idea that the unsuccessful but repeated attempted solution actually perpetuates the problem, and thus the need to get a client to do something different (rather than more of the same), is a key concept.[11]

There was a conference held back in 1993 in New Orleans in honor of John, which resulted in a nice book edited by Wendel Ray and Steve de Shazer.[12] John was also a great mentor for Steve de Shazer – it says something very good that John was so supportive even when Steve began to move in a somewhat different direction than MRI's approach. When I once interviewed John and Steve,[13] John said he wanted his lasting message to be "Stay curious." I've always appreciated Weakland's keen intelligence, his plain speaking, and his open-mindedness.

FLAVIO: You earlier mentioned that Talmon, Rosenbaum and you were presenters at the first Brief Therapy Conference. Now that more than 30 years have passed, what do you think about SST developments? How was SST seen at that time and what do you think about it now? I mean... 30 years! It's time for some consideration about its influence on the psychotherapy field. Do you think you can say something about that?

MICHAEL: Although there had been some scattered reports of one-session successes prior to our presentation in 1988 at the Brief Therapy Conference, ours was the first prospective study. It was quite controversial to suggest that someone might want to come for only one session and get benefit![14] Since then, the idea of a beneficial single session has gained more acceptance. There have been many studies demonstrating the frequency and effectiveness of SST, and there have been three international conferences – each of which resulted in the publication of a book. There was also a cover story in the July 2018 issue of *O: The Oprah Magazine*, which has a monthly readership of more than 3,000,000 people! In an interview I did a couple of years ago, I mentioned several trends that I expect will continue: more SSTs (including more walk-ins); more use of the internet; more publications, workshops, training and teaching; and more attention to cultural nuances.[15] When someone makes changes in one session, it challenges our traditional assumptions about change needing to be slow and gradual.

FLAVIO: It just came up to my mind that at our first encounter you told me you were a student of Carl Whitaker! Maybe he's not strictly a brief therapist, but he was a giant of psychotherapy. What can you tell me about him?

MICHAEL: Here's a picture. [*Michael shows Flavio a picture in his phone of Michael and Carl Whitaker in 1974*]

FLAVIO: You were, 27, right?

MICHAEL: Twenty-six or 27. One of my professors in graduate school –

FLAVIO: – graduate school was at Yale University?

MICHAEL: Right. And when I was going to go to the University of Wisconsin to do an internship, he said, "There's a very famous family therapist you should study with there. You should try to meet him. His name is Carl Whitaker." So when I went, I requested that Whitaker be my supervisor.

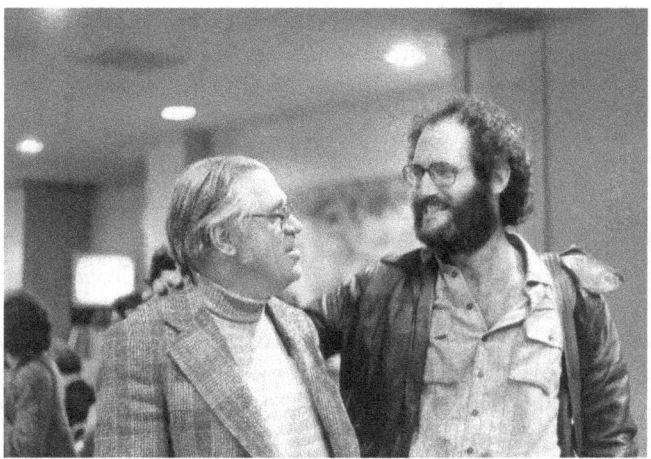

Figure 5.2 Michael with Carl Whitaker, c. 1974. ©M.F. Hoyt. Used with permission.

We met. He liked me and I liked him. He was very funny, creative, and eccentric at times. He would say things, he had a reputation for saying unusual things, but he was very organized and very smart – I think he was the chairman of his department. We could say he was "crazy like a fox."

Box 13. Carl A. Whitaker (1912–1995)

Pioneer family therapist, developer of symbolic-experiential approach. Caring and charismatic, he emphasized the importance of presence and existential responsibility and shifted the focus of therapy so that the entire family was the client.

*Quotable Quotes

1 "Every marriage is a battle between two families struggling to reproduce themselves."
2 "I deduce, therefore, that the essential objective of all psychotherapy is to get rid of the past, good and bad, and the future, good and bad, and to just *be*."
3 "*Psychopathology is proof of psychological health.* The individual who is distorted in his thinking is essentially carrying on an open war in himself rather than capitulating to the social slavery."

4 "My craziness [has given] other people the freedom to be more spontaneous, to be more intuitive, to be crazy in their own ways."

5 "Love is the anesthesia that makes the surgery possible."

*Key Publications

1 C.A. Whitaker & T.P. Malone (1953). *The Roots of Psychotherapy.* Blakiston.

2 C.A. Whitaker & A.Y. Napier (1978). *The Family Crucible.* Harper & Row.

3 C.A. Whitaker (1982). *From Psyche to System: The Evolving Therapy of Carl Whitaker* (J.R. Neill & D.P. Kniskern, Eds.). Guilford Press.

4 C.A. Whitaker & W.B. Bumberry (1988). *Dancing with the Family: A Symbolic-Experiential Approach.* Brunner/Mazel.

5 C.A. Whitaker (1989). *Midnight Musing of a Family Therapist.* (M.O. Ryan, Ed.). Norton.

6 D.V. Keith (2015). *Continuing the Experiential Approach of Carl Whitaker: Process, Practice, and Magic.* Zeig, Tucker, & Theisen.

I remember I went to his office and introduced myself and said, "I would like to be your student." We talked and he said, "Well, you know, we'll see patients together. You will be my co-therapist, we will work together." And so we saw two families. And also, once a week, I would do an intake appointment with somebody and Carl would be in the room and he would watch for an hour and then we would talk about it. Oh, lots of wonderful experiences! It's hard to summarize. I used to go sometimes to his house for dinner. I was renting a house with a roommate, a friend of mine, and I needed to build some furniture for the house, what we might call a media center for the records and the stereo equipment. Carl had a woodshop in his garage and invited me to his house to make furniture, and he would come out to the shop and help me and show me how to make it.

FLAVIO: You were very close. You were not just a teacher and his student, you were friends.

MICHAEL: He was probably 65 or something years old and he was famous, and I was an intern who was 27. We were not really friends, but he liked me. He could see that I was a good person and bright. We were friendly and I think what he did was, in a limited way, he adopted me. "Would you like to come Sunday night and have dinner with us?" he asked. "Oh yes, of course." He also lent me his skis so that I could learn how to cross-country ski. There was an assistant professor, James Gustafson, and I was just an intern and Jim taught me how to ski on Carl's borrowed skis. Now Jim is semi-retired. He still lives in Wisconsin. He is a well-known professor of psychiatry there and has written a bunch of really good books. I just recently wrote an endorsement for his new book.[16] It is funny, you know, 40 years later.

FLAVIO: Where did you live when you were with Carl Whitaker?

MICHAEL: In Madison, Wisconsin – that's where the main campus of the University of Wisconsin is located. And what I learned from Whitaker was to go to the heart of the matter, to be personal.

FLAVIO: What do you mean?

MICHAEL: His idea was to create experiences for people.[17] I remember I was asking him, "Why did you do that?" and "What did you see?" and he said, "Why? You have to do it your own way." I said, "Yes, but if I could look through your eyes for a minute, I'll see things and then I'll figure out what to do." It seems like everybody has a story about Carl Whitaker doing something crazy and eccentric, like falling asleep in a session and waking up and telling his dream to the patient. People have these funny stories. My experience was that when we would do the intake interviews, he would mostly watch to see if there was something I missed, which he would ask about at the end. But then, when the patient would leave, he would tell me "Why did you ask this and why did you ask that, and did you notice this?" and "What do you think the diagnosis is?" and "Why did you ask this question?" and "When the patient said that, did you think maybe she meant ...?" He was very sharp and very, very smart.

FLAVIO: What do you think are the differences between Erickson's and Whitaker's ways of teaching their students?

MICHAEL: When you are teaching, you're teaching something to someone. So, if the someone is already sophisticated, it's different than if you're teaching a beginner. It depends on what and who you are teaching. So, are you teaching an attitude? Or are you teaching a technique? Are you teaching how to work with a particular problem? A lot of what I was learning from Whitaker was just how to be in the room with patients and how to relate to people and how to conduct the interview. And *how to be myself.*

FLAVIO: Was he evocative like Erickson?

MICHAEL: Whitaker always wanted to bring in more and more people: "Bring your sister to the appointment, bring your next-door neighbor, bring your ex-wife as well as your wife." He was always adding people on. He had the idea that people are part of a system. I never studied with Erickson, so I don't have any direct experience to compare. I've watched a lot of the videotapes and read books, including the famous teaching seminar that Jeff Zeig[18] made a book about – they recorded Erickson telling stories about work with a client. Erickson most of the time did not explain things. He would not say: "Well, there were three techniques that I could have used and because of this..." He would just tell another story: "Well, that reminds me of a time somebody came in and..." You learned a lesson, you'd see a way to do it. He wouldn't explicitly tell you what to do.

FLAVIO: Why did Erickson do that? Why did he never just say, "You have to do this, you have to do that, use this technique"?

MICHAEL: He was a storyteller. I have seen some videotapes that almost nobody has seen – they are not available – of John Frykman interviewing Erickson.[19] John knew Erickson and they made some tapes where he would ask Erickson questions and Erickson gave regular answers: "I was thinking of this and when the guy said what he said, that's why I did that." In these unpublished tapes, he gave normal, linear explanations. Usually it was much more multileveled storytelling, and you'd be left wondering, "What does that mean? There's a message in there." I never directly experienced Erickson as a teacher. I have learned things about him, but I was never there with him. People say he would talk for hours and hours and they would begin to think, "Maybe he's talking about me?" and they'd start searching in their own experience.

FLAVIO: Some people must have been frustrated by this way of teaching: "Oh, I don't understand. He's just telling stories." I read in a book that Erickson loved to tell jokes and he loved to make quizzes, but he would not tell you the solution unless you struggled and then said you gave up.[20] Probably telling a story is the same thing: it is a way to say, "Squeeze your mind, try to find the solution, your personal interpretation." Right?

MICHAEL: Sometimes you can tell somebody the answer is "A." Other times it's better to leave it unclear and let the other person figure it out. When they say, "I think the answer is 'A,'" then that's *their* answer.

FLAVIO: What about Whitaker's way of teaching?

MCIHAEL: My experience with Whitaker is that sometimes he would be a model. You'd try to watch and see what he did. Sometimes he would explain things. I'm trying to think about an example that I wrote about.[21] A family came, and the father was having some problems. And the father's mother was coming to the appointments. There was one week where the grandmother did not come to the appointment. But the children were there, and the father and the mother were there. It was one of the (grand) children's birthdays and they brought a cake. We were going to have a cake, but the grandmother did not come. I like chocolate cake and at the end of the session, I wanted a piece of cake. Whitaker said, "No, we can sing Happy Birthday, but you have to take the cake home to grandmother, to show her that she is more important to your family than we are." It was very lovely. It got me to thinking about what it meant that the grand-mother wasn't there and how she would feel if we had celebrated without her. While I was thinking about chocolate cake, Whitaker was thinking of the system, the bigger picture. And he never said to me that we should think about the other family members and how to include them. He just did it. So I learned that we should remember that we are not part of the family. In sports we would say we are not the player, we are the coach. And so, we were trying to help their family get together instead of us becoming a member of the family.[22]

FLAVIO: I've heard you say, "We're not the golf player, we are the caddy."[23]

MICHAEL: Yes. I can think of other moments with Whitaker that were very special. Another family came in, and Whitaker said, "I will be the therapist as long as you can be with me as the co-therapist." So, I became the co-therapist – even though he did most of the work, of course. It was the first or second session, and I'm sitting there with the famous Dr. Whitaker and he's doing all these things and talking with this family. There were several children, all boys. The father was talking about how his father had died and he had gone to the father's grave – he was having some sort of crisis. And all the boys were sitting there, and they were kind of bored and acting distracted and goofy. And I leaned over and said something in the ear of the first boy and the boy's eyes got big, and he leaned over and said something to the next one and then down the line and then all the boys were listening. When they left, Whitaker asked me, "What did you say to them?" and I said, "I told the first boy, 'I know it's boring now, but pay attention: when your father dies, this will be very interesting.'" Whitaker gave me a high five. In another early session, we were there with the family. Whitaker was doing most of the talking and I'm sitting here, watching them going back and forth, and the father turned to me and challengingly said: "So, what is your role here? What do you do?" And I said, "I'm the ventriloquist."

We stayed in touch. In 1990 there was an Evolution of Psychotherapy Conference, and I spent some time with Whitaker there. It was very special.

When I first began to work at Kaiser, back in 1979, one time I was in my office in Hayward [California] and the telephone rang. I picked it up and the voice says, "This is Mark Stern. I'm the editor of the journal *Voices* and I'm calling to invite you to write an article." I said, "Huh? You're calling to invite *me* to write an article for *Voices*?" He said, "Yes, Carl Whitaker told me that you're somebody special and that I should call you."[24]

FLAVIO: Wow!

MICHAEL: Yes, it was a very sweet moment – I haven't come down yet!

I think what I learned from Whitaker is, do it your own way. Use humor or be clever or say some crazy thing. Somebody else would do it in a different way. He was encouraging me to find my own way to do therapy, but I had to have a reason for what I was doing – there should be a purpose, what we're calling a "logic."[25] When we're a young professional we need a guide, a mentor, a hero, a teacher. They're not just the teacher like a professor – a mentor helps you become confident in yourself and that inspires you. I think for Jay Haley that was Erickson, and I think for Steve de Shazer that was John Weakland. Somebody comes along and says, "You have skill and you can be special." It doesn't have to be somebody famous. I think that's what Whitaker was for me and what Bob Goulding was for me also in a different way. But, after some time you have to say, "Okay, but I'm not going to be Carl Whitaker." I'm going to be myself: Michael Hoyt or Flavio Cannistrà or Joe Smith or Federico Piccirilli[26]. And so Whitaker's message was "Use yourself. Make a difference, and do it your own way."

FLAVIO: So, we could say "Humor is not a technique, *you* are."

MICHAEL: Yes. I wasn't yet 30 years old. It's different from now when I am 70 years old. If somebody walks in and there's a tall man with dark hair, a kind of handsome young man, you're going to relate to him differently compared to seeing a guy with white hair, who is half bald and he's 65 or 70 years old. That guy seems maybe like your uncle or your grandfather. You have to use whoever you are at that time.

FLAVIO: I think it is quite normal that a young professional, a young psychologist in the early days of his career tries to be like someone, looks for a model. I think it is also important to have a mentor, or somebody, or your own experience, to help you to be yourself. To say, "Okay, you have followed a model, but now it is time to find your way!"

Who is another underappreciated great?

MICHAEL: Bob and Mary Goulding. I met Bob Goulding at that first Evolution of Psychotherapy Conference in 1985. I fell in love with Bob because he was so human and he was funny and he was down to earth. And after he gave his presentation, I went up to him and I said, "What would I learn if I come to your training?" And he said [*lowering his voice to sound like Goulding*], "Well, that depends on what you do," sort of putting the responsibility on me. And normally I would think about it for a couple of years and never do it. But instead, I went home and I called the Gouldings, found out how much, mailed them a check and signed up to do a training. They lived in Watsonville, California, south of San Francisco. And they had an institute, the Western Institute for Group and Family Therapy. I did a training for a week. And then I did another training. After I did the second training, my wife said to me: "When you came back, you seemed more normal than you have ever been. Usually you go to one of these trainings, you come back and you're talking in some weird way with new words, have different ways of thinking and acting and it's all strange, but now you seem very present and real." And I told her what had happened. And then Jennifer and I went together, I forget if it was for one week or two weeks. We lived there. We did it every day, all day long. We made friends. A couple of the people I'm still friends with. At the Brief Therapy Conference we were just at, there was a woman who was there 30 years ago. I had not seen her in 30 years! And I saw her at the Brief Therapy Conference. She was pregnant when we were at the training and now she has a daughter who's an adult. We were talking. It was a wonderful kind of connection to see her again.

Box 14. Robert L. Goulding (1917–1992) and Mary McClure Goulding (1925–2008)

Developers of Redecision Therapy, an integration of Transactional Analysis and Gestalt Therapy plus their own innovations. Their model emphasized both assisting the client to make redecisions to overcome limiting beliefs and getting the client to *take action*, not just to increase awareness or understanding.

*Quotable Quotes

1 "In our experience most good therapy is centered on assisting the patient to break through a series of impasses, which had their origins in messages he received in childhood and decisions he made about those messages. As the patient works through his impasses, we offer cognitive understanding of how his archaic patterns of thinking, feeling, and doing fit together and affect his life in the present."

2. "WHAT ARE YOU WILLING TO CHANGE TODAY?" (Goulding & Goulding Contract Question). Each element is important:
    What (specificity, goal, target, focus)
    are (active verb, present tense)
    you (self as agent, personal function)
    willing (choice, responsibility, initiative)
    to change (alter or modify, not just "work on," "try," "talk about," "explore" or "understand")
    today (now, in the moment)
    ? (inquiry, open field, therapist inviting and respectfully receptive but not insistent)

3. "The first con in each session is tremendously important because, if it is not confronted, the entire session may be devoted to acting out the con [...] A con, delivered in the first session, may set the stage for the entire course of treatment, if not confronted."

4. "Redecision is a beginning rather than an ending. After redecision, the person begins to think, feel, and behave in new ways. At this point he may decide to terminate therapy. We applaud this choice. Our philosophy of treatment is that therapy should be as condensed and quick as possible and that termination is a triumph, like graduation."

5. "Short-term therapy requires a skillful therapist. To help the client effect personal changes in the shortest possible time, the therapist must work precisely and efficiently, focusing only on material that is

relevant to the contract. [...] I am impressed with the fact that clients continue to make important changes after therapy has ended, if they have learned to believe in their own ability to change their lives."

*Key Publications

1 R.L. Goulding & M.M. Goulding (1978). *The Power Is in the Patient.* TA Press.
2 M.M. Goulding & R.L. Goulding (1979). *Changing Lives through Redecision Therapy.* Brunner/Mazel.
3 M.M. Goulding (1985). *Who's Been Living in Your Head?* (rev. ed.). WIGFT Press.
4 M.M. Goulding & R.L. Goulding (1989). *Not to Worry! How to Free Yourself from Unnecessary Anxiety and Channel Your Worries into Positive Action.* William Morrow.
5 M.M. Goulding (1996). *A Time to Say Goodbye: Moving Beyond Loss.* Papier-Mache Press.

But back to Bob and Mary Goulding. Mary even wrote a paper called "Getting the Important Work Done Fast,"[27] and she said the important work is to make an alliance, find out the client's goal, what they're willing to do to achieve it – and assist them to make the appropriate redecision. So they would ask a specific question: "What are you willing to change today?" Not just what do you want to talk about, what do you want to explore, but what are you willing to do differently, *What are you willing to change today?* And so it was very focused. They called this the *contract*, the goal, and then they developed the technology.

What I learned from them the most was to focus therapy and to be active, not just say, "What does that remind you of? How do you feel? What else? Oh, it sounds like you have a lot of ideas," but to actually help the client look at things differently in a very active way. I also learned from Bob and from Mary, the importance of being responsible, autonomous. That when people say, "You *made* me feel..." nobody *makes* you feel any way unless they actually hit you. They may encourage you to feel that way. They may threaten you, they may want you to feel that way, they may attempt to entice or provoke you, but you have some choice about how you feel. So, the idea of confidence, control, choice – that you're responsible for your existence – I learned a lot of that from Bob and Mary.

FLAVIO: Why did you choose them when I asked you?

MICHAEL: Because they were brilliant and wonderful and mean a lot to me.[28]
They were my teachers and they are being forgotten because almost nobody

talks anymore about Transactional Analysis or even Gestalt therapy. No one talks about Eric Berne and T.A. and "I'm OK, You're OK." All of that is sort of ancient history, and I think there are very good things to learn. By the way, that phrase, "I'm OK, You're OK," Bob Goulding actually invented that phrase one morning while talking with Eric Berne.[29]

Bob Goulding had trained in psychodynamic therapy. So did Mary. Then they learned Gestalt therapy with Fritz Perls. He and Fritz Perls were close, and Bob and Mary learned theory from Eric Berne. But then, they put it together to make it more action-oriented therapy where people would have a new experience. I once realized in one of the workshops, and Bob agreed with me, I said: "Explanation leads to recognition, and experience leads to change." If you explain something (like "Oh, you're doing this because your mother treated you that way" or "You're co-dependent, or you're anxious, or you're...") you get an explanation, you may recognize it; but then you need to have a new experience. So their therapy was much more experiential. It wasn't just talking about things but doing something differently to have a new experience. When you have the new experience, you can have a new result, a new outcome: "Oh, I was scared that if I spoke up, everybody would hate me, but I spoke up and nothing bad happened. So now I can see it's safe, at least with some people, to express myself. Maybe not with everybody. I have to be careful, but I can speak up."

Bob and Mary were on the faculty of the first Evolution of Psychotherapy Conference in 1985. They also were on the faculty for the second Evolution Conference in 1990. In 1990, however, Bob was sick. He had COPD, chronic obstructive pulmonary disease. He was a heavy smoker. He drank also, and he had a lot of coughing and health problems. And so he was not able to go to the conference. I went to the conference. Mary was there and every day at the end of the day I would go to my hotel room and I would call Bob and for an hour I would tell him about the conference. First he would ask me, "How did Mary do, what happened, tell me about it." And I'd tell him about Mary's work, her presentations, and what people said. And then I would tell him about other things and we would discuss it.

Near the end of Bob's life, Bob had a lot of health problems and he still smoked a lot of cigarettes, but he could not drink anymore. He could not sleep. His body was a mess. He was in terrible condition. And one day we were sitting talking and I said, "Bob, it really bothers me that you are smoking. You should not be smoking. You're sick, you're old, you should not be smoking." And Bob said to me straight out, "Michael, I can no longer have sex. I can barely go to the toilet." He went through the list. He said, "My only pleasure now is smoking cigarettes. So, if you say one more negative thing about cigarettes, I don't want to be your friend. This is my last pleasure." And I looked at him and I said, "I have one thing I would like to say." He said, "What is it?" And I reached over and I picked up the lighter. I said, "Can I light a cigarette for you?" And he smiled. And then

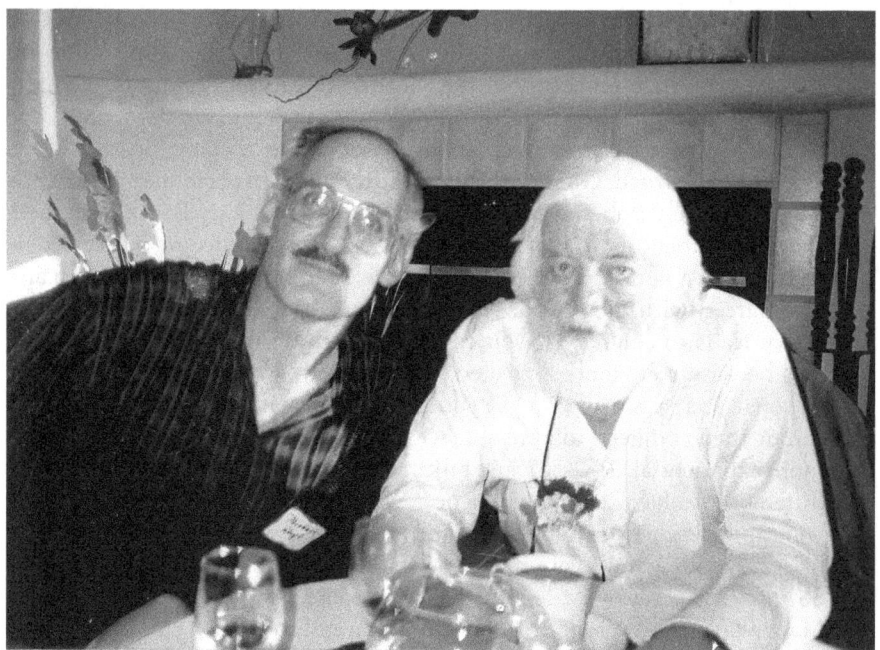

Figure 5.3 Michael with Bob Goulding, c. 1991. ©M.F. Hoyt. Used with permission.

we lit a cigarette and I think I smoked one with him. And I realized it was very important that he have his pleasure. And he said, "I appreciate you're worried about me. But you know, I'm old, I'm sick. I'm not going to be around much longer, so let me have what I want without a hassle."

Bob was very interested in sports. One day I was going to go play golf nearby when I was staying there at the Western Institute. I had my golf clubs. He said, "How are you going to do?" And I said, "Oh, I'm going to try to break 90." He said, "Break 80." And I said, "Let's be realistic. I'm not that good. I break 90, I'll be happy." I think I made an 82 or 83 that day.

Then, at almost the very end of his life, an interesting thing happened. I was at home in Mill Valley and the telephone rang and it was Mary and she said, "Michael, Bob is in the hospital. He's going to die in the next couple of days. If you want to come and see him, you have to come now." I got right in my car and I drove two hours to Santa Cruz where he was in the hospital. When I went in, Mary was there. She was with Bob. He had oxygen, and he wasn't very well. She said, "Maybe you want to talk for a few minutes, I'm going to go for a walk." She left Bob and me alone, to be together. We had a very beautiful, very personal talk. I loved him. He loved me. We were friends, he was my teacher. I was his student, but he also treated me like a professional. We finally – we said our goodbye. I kissed him on the cheek. "I love you." "I love you." "Thank you." "God bless you." And I left – and he did not die! He got better, not because of me, but somehow he got better and he got to go home for a couple of months. And so when I went and saw him, I thought I'd said my goodbye. It was very weird because I drove home with tears in my eyes and he was going to die and I said goodbye to my teacher. And then a couple of days later I called Mary. "How's Bob?" I thought she might say he was dead. And she said, "He's going home. His breathing got better." So he went home and then I went and saw him a couple of times. And then eventually he died, and we had a big ceremony, a hundred people came and we talked about Bob. We sang *Amazing Grace*. We had a good time. We all held hands in a big circle and we went around for hours and told stories about Bob. Funny stories, sad stories, good stories. Patients were there, family was there, the Western Institute staff were there, the cook was there, his doctor was there, lots of people came. He was one of those special people. He was very, very, very intelligent and very down to earth. He had done a general practice as a medical doctor in South Dakota or North Dakota before he went back to become a psychiatrist. He liked being in people's lives. He loved helping people. He loved jazz music. He was a character, and he was one of those people, when he would talk to you, you would always feel good.

He was one of those people that made you feel special, that you're good, you're smart, you could do things. He brought out the best in people. He was very loving and kind. I had a patient, she went to see Bob. She had cerebral palsy, when you're born you don't get enough oxygen so it makes you uncoordinated. Your speech can be difficult. Her intelligence was fine, but she talked kind of like this *{makes his voice tremble}* and her voice would break, and if she had a tremor, she would shake. So I said, "Maybe you should go visit Dr. Goulding, I think he could help you." And she went to one of their residential conferences for a week and she said the day she met him, it changed her life. What happened was, she walked in, it took her a little bit to walk up the stairs. She was young, she was in her 30s, she walked in and she went up, and he was sitting at the table watching television and she said, "Oh, hello, Dr. Goulding" and with her trembling voice introduced herself. "Michael sent me. Oh, I want you to know that I have CP, cerebral palsy," and Goulding said, "I can see that you shake and I can hear your voice, but I am much more interested in finding out who you are." And her whole life changed. She said, she became a person who had CP, instead of CP had her. "I'm a valuable person *and* I've got this problem, but it's not going to be my identity. I should not introduce myself as 'I have CP,' I should say, 'Hi, my name is _____,' say my name and all that." That was a very typical Goulding moment.

Bob Goulding was the best therapist I ever saw. He, with everybody he worked, somehow always knew what to do. I don't know how he did it. Sometimes he would be gentle, sometimes he would be very confronting. He would say different things, but with everybody he was very good. Mary Goulding was very, very good, also, and there are other very good therapists. But Bob – in baseball we say, "You hit a home run." Well, Bob always hit a home run. I don't know how he did it. I would sit and I would watch him for hours and hours with clients, and on videotapes, and doing our training. And then at night I would sit with him smoking cigarettes, and I would ask him different questions about "Why did you do this?" why he did that, how did he know to do what he did? And he was just so good. I think they both were. They were also very good friends with Virginia Satir and with the people called Erving and Miriam Polster – they were the best of the Gestalt people. They also knew Albert Ellis, and they all had some of the same ideas about responsibility and seeing what you could do differently and that you're not controlled by your circumstances: You make the choice. Jeff Zeig had trained with them. When we had the memorial funeral service for Mary, Jeff was there, and other people: Muriel James who wrote *Born to Win* and *It's Never Too Late to Be Happy*, and Ellyn Bader who is a very well-known and excellent couple therapist, she trained with Bob and Mary.[30]

FLAVIO: Your relationship with them, it seems to me that there was a difference from the relationship you had with Carl Whitaker.

MICHAEL: I was younger when I met Carl Whitaker, I was 26 or 27. I wasn't 38. One time I gave a presentation at the Gouldings' Western Institute. And Bob insisted on paying me $100. I said, "You don't have to pay me" and he said, "No, you're a professional and because you're a professional, you should expect to be paid." So I accepted the money and it was very symbolic. He was sort of ratifying or signifying that I'm somebody that should be paid for what I do. He had written a paper about fishing and catching fish[31] and he looked at me and he said, "Michael, the paper about fishing is not really about fish." I said, "It's not?" And he looked at me: "No, it's about getting things, earning things with hard work and skill."

FLAVIO: In a way, Bob seems to me really Ericksonian.

MICHAEL: Well, he was evocative. He also had his Redecision theory, a T.A. theory, Parent-Adult-Child and put them in a chair and talk to them. And they had ideas about how we get stuck: we're being too adaptive, we're not being true to ourselves. He was different than Erickson. He did not use formal hypnosis. But he had the idea that people had a lot more ability.

I remember once, I was sort of shocked, we were at a training session and some woman in the group started to cry and some other woman jumped up with a box of Kleenex; she was going to go over and Bob said to the second woman, "Sit down. Don't give her the Kleenex. She does this every time. This is just a game she does to get attention." And I thought, "How mean and how cruel. How could you say that?" And then it turned out, of course, he was right. This was a way for her to get attention for trouble instead of growing up and being more healthy. She got better. I never saw him do that again. I don't mean to say that he was mean. Not at all. He was very loving toward people.

Bob could certainly talk intellectually and theoretically, but Bob liked to not act like he was showing off. He was just sort of himself. When they had the first Brief Therapy Conference, it was in 1988 in San Francisco and one night I had a party at my house. I invited some people and Bob and Mary came to the party and there were other people at the party, there was Moshe Talmon, there was Steve de Shazer, and Yvonne Dolan, and Hans Strupp and Nick Cummings, and some others. Bob and Mary were there and I spent most of the evening sitting and talking with Bob outside on the patio because he wanted to smoke cigarettes and didn't want to smoke in the house. I remember Bob said to me, "Michael, you should go be with your other guests." I said, "Bob, I wanted you to be here. Everyone else, I'll talk to another time." I just loved Bob. I was very glad to know Bob, to see Bob. It was a blessing because he was much older. He got sick, he died. When I went to the 1985 Evolution of Psychotherapy Conference, that first time I saw him, I could have gone and seen somebody else for that hour, you know, or somebody could have said, "Oh, let's go have a cup of coffee" and I would have missed it. I think some of what we do, we do deliberately and we're also blessed or lucky or fortunate.

I think that Bob and Mary were very special. After Bob died, Mary moved to San Francisco for a couple of years, and then she sold the place in San Francisco and she was living half the year in Cuba and also in California where her children lived. Mary and I had been talking on the telephone and I was going to go to teach with her in Cuba. And there was a Brief Therapy Conference, and I walked in and there was a big picture of Mary on the wall. I smiled and then somebody came up and they said, "Michael, do you know that Mary died last month?" "Oh, no." She had died. She had very bad diabetes and she had other health problems, and she died and so I never got to go to Cuba with Mary, unfortunately.

Here is something Mary did; this is very Mary. In Japan, sometimes when a samurai was going to die, they would give him a piece of paper and a pen so that he could write a last poem as an expression of his entire life. So, when Mary got very sick, she was home (in San Francisco) and she called 911. They advised her to unlock the door so the paramedics and the ambulance could get in, which she did, but she knew she would not survive and she took a piece of paper and she wrote a last letter to all of her friends before she died. Her dying breath kind of idea. She wrote: "No matter when I died there would be places left to visit and beauty still to enjoy. I cannot imagine a better life than I have had. Many thanks and much much love to all of you." A blow-up of the note was on the wall, with her photo. It was very sweet. I put it as an epigraph in the front of the book *Therapist Stories of Inspiration, Passion, and Renewal*.

Another thing about Bob. When we were doing the training, Bob believed that people should be responsible for themselves. *Autonomy*, he called it. Not "*You* made me do it," or "Oh, I'm going to *try* to do this" meaning if someone says they are going to "try" they won't really do it. So, Bob had this big cowbell, a bell for cows, by his chair. He would pick it up and he would ring it whenever someone said "try" or "they made me." It was horrible. It was embarrassing, but it was funny and the first time you would say, "Well, I'm going to try to work on it," the bell would ring. The other day when I saw that person at the Brief Therapy Conference, I was saying something to her and I said, "I can still hear the goddamn cowbell," and she laughed and said, "I can hear it, too!" Whenever I say "I'm going to do something" and don't mean I'm really going to do it, I hear the bell ring, like Bob's saying, "Tell the truth – be honest." Everybody who was there, if I now just said "the cowbell," everybody would laugh.

FLAVIO: Tell me a little more about Mary.

MICHAEL: I'll tell you an interesting story about Mary. She went to high school in Hayward, California, and after high school she wanted to learn Spanish, so she moved to Mexico City. She was 18 or 19 years old. She decided, "I'll go live in Mexico, I'll learn Spanish." And when she was there, every day she went to where Diego Rivera was painting and she watched Rivera paint and she got to know him. So, I said to Mary one day, "Were you his girlfriend?" and she smiled and she said, "I will not tell." But I noticed on the bookshelf there were a couple of drawings, nice drawings that Diego Rivera had done and he had written in Spanish "to Mary from Diego." She was adventurous. When she came back to the United States, she became a social worker and then was very interested in psychiatric stuff and got training. And then she met Bob and then Fritz Perls.

Bob and I did an interview for hours on a video. We made it into an article that was published in the *TA Journal*. It's also reprinted in that book *Interviews with Brief Therapy Experts*. It has a lot of nice things in it. He would compliment my wife and I would compliment his wife. There's a lot about Bob and Mary's ideas. Bob was supervising me, and there's also another paper that we published by Hoyt and Goulding.[32] It's about T.A. and countertransference. It's a good article, but I think he also did it to support me.

Bob was old, I don't know exactly how old he was, but he was sick and he knew he wasn't gonna live a long time. Wow, I just understood why I played that Warren Zevon song, *Keep Me in Your Heart*, on the car CD while we were driving. As you get older, you want to pass on whatever benefits you have had – at least some people do. I was very lucky. I got Carl Whitaker, and then Bob and Mary, and later I knew some others. I got to know Haley, and Steve de Shazer and Insoo, and I got to know Michael White a bit.

FLAVIO: I want to ask you about Steve and Insoo.

MICHAEL: Sure. I was fortunate to spend time with them and actually published a couple of papers with them.[33] We also visited in one another's homes and once spent a week together in Japan. I met them when Moshe Talmon introduced us at the 1988 Brief Therapy Conference. I liked them both, a lot. They were very different – Steve was an introverted minimalist – sometimes he seemed to look at things almost like a visitor from another planet, so he saw things with a certain clarity. He also was an excellent cook, played the saxophone, loved baseball and the Milwaukee Braves and really appreciated Sherlock Holmes – indeed, Steve was a "solution detective."

Insoo was much warmer and vivacious – I called her my "Seoul sister" (she was born in Seoul, Korea) – we joked around and sent funny emails back and forth. I was very sad when they passed away, first Steve in 2005 and then within a year or so, Insoo. The folks at BRIEF (formerly the Brief Therapy Practice) in London – Chris Iveson, Harvey Ratner, and Evan George – are, in my humble opinion, the keepers of the flame and the best proponents of SFBT. They were close with Steve and Insoo, and I'm sure Steve and Insoo would be pleased to see how the London group has refined SFBT.

I recall it was around 1990 when Scott Miller, who was still affiliated with the Brief Family Therapy Center in Milwaukee, came to San Rafael, California (near where I live) and taught an excellent workshop on SFBT. It was, for me, a very positive "fork in the road." Scott and I wound up coauthoring a paper, by the way.[34] Of course, even before the Miracle Question, Alfred Adler had talked about waving a magic wand and asking clients what would be different and better. The story about the origins of the Miracle Question is quoted in my 2009 book.[35]

FLAVIO: Thank you, Michael, for sharing this. It's interesting to know the people behind the therapists – you can learn more about the therapy, the theory, its strengths and its limits. Please continue a little about de Shazer and Berg.

MICHAEL: What I know about the people behind the different theories is, they are people. They're all smart and they all, you know, care about people. They all work very hard.

FLAVIO: When I think of your book, *Some Stories Are Better than Others*, it came in my mind, the title, "some persons are better than others."

MICHAEL: Well, whatever "better" means. Some people are kinder, some people are more helpful. Some people are smarter. Honest and ethical count for a lot, too.

In 1988, the Brief Therapy Conference was in San Francisco and I was standing in the lobby of the hotel talking to Moshe Talmon, and Moshe said, "Oh, there's Steve de Shazer." Moshe had gone to Milwaukee and had done something with Steve. And I was planning to have a party at my house, and I said, "Should I invite him to the party?" And Moshe said,

"Yeah, of course." So I invited Steve to the party. Steve was standing there and I said, "Oh, we're having a party in a couple days at my house. If you could come, it'd be good. We'll have food, a nice evening, we're having some people." And Steve said, "Okay, I'll come, and so will..." and he pointed to five different people he was with, "Oh, and this person, too." And he invited all these people! Suddenly I thought, "Oh my God, you just invited all those people. I don't have enough food. And I wasn't planning on all those people. I thought I was inviting you and now I've got more people." And it was a little awkward, but it turned out the people he invited, several of them I know very well now and it was all very good. But I met Steve through Moshe that time. But I was mostly hanging out with Bob Goulding.

FLAVIO: Ok, it was *that* party!

MICHAEL: Yes, it was *that* party, and Bob was there and Mary was there. Mary liked it, she said, "You always have the best food at parties." The Gouldings were there and a man named Hans Strupp, who was very well known in the short-term psychodynamic world.[36] He was very good, had a lot to say. And Nick Cummings came, and later I got to know Cummings more and a couple of other people.

I had read *Clues* and *Keys*[37] and I talked to de Shazer that evening, but not a lot. But then, a couple of years later, Scott Miller came to California to give a presentation. It was in San Rafael, near where I live, and he came to give a workshop about solution-focused therapy and talked about the Miracle Question and scaling questions and coping questions, the different kinds of questions. The workshop with Scott was really good and I learned a bunch. I liked it a lot. And then I wrote a paper and I sent it to Scott and Scott wrote back to me – I may be putting this together in time a little too close, but I think it was right after that. I sent him this paper and he wrote back, saying, "Michael, thank you for the paper. But when I read the paper, I feel like the way you're writing it, you're saying either 'Agree with me, or you are wrong' instead of saying 'Here's my way of thinking and you may have others.' You're saying, 'This is the right way.'"

And he said, "You're stimulating resistance." When I read Scott's reply, I said, "You're wrong!" *{laughs}* And then I thought about it – "He's a nice guy, he's smart" – and I had a look at it again, and you know, he was right! I could see that. And it changed the way I write. It changed the way I think. I offer things now instead of forcing them. I try to make it attractive, instead of winning an argument all the time. Scott has developed in different directions and is doing different things, he's no longer teaching SFBT, but Scott was part of my really getting interested in solution-focused therapy, very much so.

FLAVIO: What about Steve?

MICHAEL: Steve was, we might say in English, a bit of an "odd duck" or a strange person. He was quiet. He was a little socially awkward. He wasn't

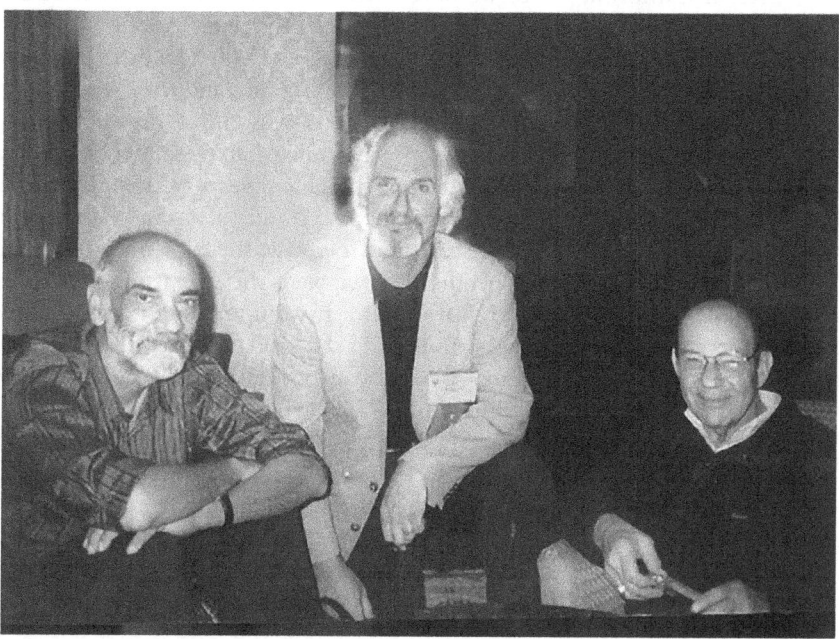

Figure 5.4 Michael (middle) with Steve de Shazer (left) and Richard ("Dick") Fisch (right), c. 1994. ©M.F. Hoyt. Used with permission.

gregarious, he wasn't a big talker. He had studied at MRI with Paul Watzlawick, John Weakland, and Dick Fisch, and that's where he met Insoo.

He was brilliant and he was a very kind, nice man. But because he didn't talk a lot, he would sort of be on the outside. He'd watch how things would happen. Steve was interested in Sherlock Holmes' detective stories. Steve was an expert saxophone player. He loved music, had different interests. He liked Wittgenstein a lot. One of the ways Steve and I connected was through baseball. Steve grew up near Milwaukee and was a big fan of the Milwaukee baseball team. And I knew who his favorite pitcher was. And so, when I went to the Baseball Hall of Fame, I got a picture of his favorite player and mailed it to him. He liked that. And he loved to cook. So Steve and I, we got to be friendly.

And then, I got invited to go to Japan. Maybe Insoo had something to do with that. She probably did. I was going to be a speaker in Japan. I took my son Alex with – he loves Japan – and when I went to Japan, Insoo was there. Insoo was Korean; she was born near Seoul. And Steve was there in Japan, and some other people. Bill O'Hanlon and Mary Goulding were there. I forget who else was there.

I live in California where we have earthquakes and there had been an earthquake in Japan, in Kobe, a very bad earthquake. And I was very moved, I could see how horrible it was, people were killed and the Japanese people who were inviting us, they were very, very nice and they were going to pay us a bunch of money. So I sent a letter to some of my colleagues, saying maybe we should give some money to help Japanese mental-health services during the recovery from the earthquake. Everyone thought that'd be a nice thing. So we donated some money. I said to Insoo, "Can we do this?" and she said, "Let me take care of it" because, she explained, it would be too embarrassing for the people that we were the guests of if we gave them money. It wouldn't be right for them. It would make them feel awkward where they should be honoring us. So she kind of helped this happen. And somebody met me and my son at the airport and took very good care of us. Insoo would ask me things like, "Oh, what is your son into?" and I'd say, "He's interested in martial arts" and she'd ask, "Oh, and what else do you like to do?" Somebody took us to a Kendo lesson, the martial art. We went to somebody's house for dinner and we stayed there. And then they took us and we walked from one village to another in the mountains. They were very, very, very kind to us. I learned a lot of things. One thing was culturally, how polite and courteous Japanese people are. And how you don't show off.

One day I was standing in the center of the plaza, in Kyoto, and there were a thousand people and they're all rushing. People had lots of bicycles. Nobody was yelling and nobody was honking their horn or ringing their bell. Everybody paid attention to everybody, how it all worked together. And I got the idea of truly being systemic, being collective and being part of a bigger organization. Americans, we're very independent. Everyone for themselves, you know, and standing in the square in Kyoto I could see how everybody was together and cooperative – this is something I learned from Insoo and the Japanese.

FLAVIO: From what you said, Insoo seems to me quite different from Steve.

MICHAEL: Insoo was much more social than Steve. We became friends. We wrote a paper together, and did some other things. I interviewed Steve and Insoo for a book and I interviewed Steve and Weakland for another book.[38] We have an expression in English. It comes, I suppose, from African-American culture, when somebody says "soul brother" or "soul sister," or "You've got soul." So I used to joke and call Insoo my "Seoul sister," because she was from Seoul, Korea, but "soul" meaning we were connected. When we went to the conference in Japan, you know, she and I were hanging out. She would send me emails when they'd be traveling. We would call each other and tell each other jokes. She was much more attuned to public relations and being social. Steve was more quiet, and very intellectual and thoughtful; they were both very nice people.

FLAVIO: They decided not to put a trademark on solution-focused.

MICHAEL: It's an orientation and it's a way of looking, looking for a solution. We're focusing on strengths, but they did not want to make it "de Shazer and Berg Therapy."

FLAVIO: It's an "open source."

MICHAEL: It's open especially because of what it is. If you're saying the client has the answer and the client is the expert, then you cannot make it about you. You have to make it about them.

FLAVIO: They didn't decide to give licenses. You know what I mean? That's pretty cool.

MICHAEL: Steve, in the late 1970s, was a psychiatric social worker and very interested in therapy and brief therapy and I think he may have met Milton Erickson once or twice and he knew Haley. So Steve went to MRI, Mental Research Institute. And Steve was studying strategic therapy and Insoo was there and that's how they met. They became friends, and husband and wife, and also business partners. They moved to Milwaukee and started the Brief Family Therapy Center in 1978.

Insoo told me a story. I have to think about how to say it. Insoo was very offended when people would be insulting either because they were racist or they would talk to women in a bad way. Some people have the attitude that if you're not white, or if you have an accent, you must not be smart. In addition to English and Korean, Insoo spoke some German and some French, and some Japanese, and maybe some other languages. She was very educated, very very smart and very sophisticated. And she deliberately developed a therapy that would focus on seeing the strengths that people had.

FLAVIO: What was the difference between Steve's way to do the therapy and Insoo's way?

MICHAEL: Steve was like a surgeon or Zen master.

FLAVIO: What do you mean?

MICHAEL: He was very precise. If you'd watch Insoo, she'd effusively say [*raises voice to sound like Insoo*], "Wow, how did you do that? Oh, you love your husband! Really? Oh, does he know how much you love him?" She had a persona that Steve called "Insoo the Incredulous." Like "Wow" – she couldn't believe it, you know? And Weakland was "Weakland the Dense," like he would play that he was dumb, that he didn't understand. He would do the one-down: "Oh, help me understand this – how do you do that?" And he was very, very smart. Yeah, they had their different personalities, but they all had the idea: look for strengths and solutions.

de Shazer, when he was at MRI, was very good at defining and developing strategies.[39] He was very clever. And then one day he realized, "You know, we don't need all the strategies. It's too hard on the therapist. You don't have to be brilliant. You don't have to outsmart the patient. Just find out when the patient is doing better, what are they doing? Get them to do more of it. I don't have to outsmart the patient." So that was the death of resistance. People resist you if you're trying to make them do something they don't want to do. Resistance was the idea that the therapist has to conquer the patient.

FLAVIO: I see.

MICHAEL: So, they were different. Very different.

FLAVIO: de Shazer wrote 4 or 5 books.

MICHAEL: Yeah.

FLAVIO: And then he stopped writing books. He continued to write articles but he stopped writing books. Why?

MICHAEL: I think he said what he wanted to say. He died in 2005.

FLAVIO: Insoo died in 2006.

MICHAEL: Right. de Shazer died first. And Insoo died a year later. de Shazer died on September 11, 2005, in Vienna.

FLAVIO: Seriously? That was my 24th birthday!

MICHAEL: He was sick. He had some kind of blood problem. I don't think it was leukemia, but it was something. His skin looked unhealthy.

FLAVIO: Did you ever attend some of Steve's trainings?

MICHAEL: I went to one for two days. He was doing it in San Francisco. He was doing it for the California School of Professional Psychology. I said, "I know him. Would you like me to be his host? I'll meet him at the airport." They said, "Oh yeah, sure." So, we spent a couple of days doing that. I did not do a lot of training with him. I read all the books and I would talk to him about things sometimes. We would talk about sports and music, and when I was going to go to China I said, "Do you have any advice?" And he said, "Yeah, there should be good food." He also said, "My advice is bring a nice present for your translator because you want them to like you." I said, "Oh, that's very good advice."

FLAVIO: It seems that everyone taught you something useful for your life.

MICHAEL: I have a tendency to doubt myself and to be unsure. And what they all did is they told me I was very smart and if I would just be myself it would be good, that I didn't have to be something else. I think that's the ultimate thing I got from all of them: "You're good, you're okay, we approve." That's a good word, "approve."

FLAVIO: If you have to think about something particular, something special, about Steve and/or Insoo –

MICHAEL: – what do I think they would say?

FLAVIO: No, no. If you think about something that you bring from them, Insoo and/or Steve, what would be?

MICHAEL: From them – The Miracle Question. But not even just the question, but rather looking for where the clients want to go, looking for the positive outcome instead of talking about the problem. That's what I got.

FLAVIO: That's a big change.

MICHAEL: A big change. I went from problem focus to solution focus. I think that's the main thing from them. I think the idea of having a goal, I got from the Gouldings, and the client having power and responsibility, I got from the Gouldings. But solution focus, I got more of that from Steve and Insoo. Paying attention to language from all of them. Actually, somebody watching me probably would not be able to say what kind of therapist I am. "Are you solution-focused? Are you cognitive-behavioral? You seem like you kind of try to encourage people." But I'm not a classic. I don't often ask scaling questions. I seldom ask the Miracle Question. I usually don't say, "What are your best hopes for today's meeting?" I do give compliments: "Hey, you're good at that. You're smart." I think I have my own way of doing things.

FLAVIO: In one interview with Steve you say "PTSD," and Steve said –

MICHAEL: [*quoting*] – "I don't know what that is. I don't know what it is." He was serious.

FLAVIO: It's a way to say, "I don't care about labels"?

MICHAEL: I think it was "borderline personality," not PTSD, or maybe it was "MPD."[40] I think mostly it was to say, "I don't care about labels. What actually goes on with the person? 'Oh, I can't stop thinking about this, so I'm nervous about that, or I avoid certain situations, or...'" I think it was mostly to say, "Don't use the label. Tell me what really is going on." He did not think in terms of diagnoses, anxiety, depression, or even what problem are you having. It was more: "What do you want help with? What do you want? How would it be different?" He would say, "How will we know when we can stop meeting like this? What will be better so that you don't feel you need to come to therapy?" "Oh, when I go to bed and don't have a nightmare" or "I can have sex and enjoy it," or "When I can speak in public without having a panic attack" or "I can be around people and don't get drunk," you know, whatever the thing was. So he would not say, "Oh, do you have sexual dysfunction? Do you have alcoholism? Do you have anxiety disorders – generalized anxiety or a phobia?" He would just ask, "What's the specifics?" Because that was closer to where he wanted to work. William Blake, the English poet a couple of centuries ago, said we have to focus on details. Generalities are for scoundrels. Liars use them to hide things.[41] Big generalities, like saying "resistance" if they did not like what you said. So they don't want to do it. "Oh, okay. What would you like to do instead?" It's keeping it "experience-close," as the phenomenologists would say.

FLAVIO: Yes. In my way of working with clients, it's hard to see such a thing as resistance.

MICHAEL: A better word for resistance is "feedback." Feedback. So, they're telling you "I don't like that" or "That doesn't fit for me" or "I'm not ready for that." You're trying to get them to do something they don't want to do. So we say pejoratively, "they're resisting." Yeah. Well, "*Vive la résistance!*" Good. The resistance means they're controlling their space. I was once asked to go to the hospital to see a patient who was sort of depressed. He had had an operation. So I went in and introduced myself: "Hi. I'm Dr. Hoyt, I want to talk to you. I'm from the Psychiatry Department and so…" He cut me off: "Get the hell out of my room," he said. "But I'm supposed to come and help you." "I don't need any help. Just leave." So when I went back to the referrer, I said "The patient is now active and in charge. He woke up. He's back on his game."

Because of your theory, you try to direct the person in a certain way: "You have to talk about what happened. You won't get better unless you tell me what happened and cry a lot." It's my method and my method comes from my theory, my mindset. My theory tells me what I'm supposed to do. Sometimes the theory is very good, if a person wants to do it.

I'd also like to briefly give a shout-out to three others. They're all well known.

FLAVIO: Sure.

MICHAEL: The first is Bill O'Hanlon – I always learn something when I hear Bill talk or read his books.[42] In addition to ideas about doing therapy, many years ago, when I was first starting to be a presenter, Bill was very supportive, answering my questions about arrangements with sponsors, contracts and so forth. One time when I was thanking him, I politely asked why he was being so helpful and generous, and he said: "When I asked Dr. [Milton] Erickson how to rise in the profession, he told me, 'Pull up good people with you.'" Very nice! And now I'm in what the other famous Erikson, Erik Erikson, called the *generativity* phase of the life cycle[43] – trying to help deserving younger colleagues, like you.

FLAVIO: Thank you!

MICHAEL: You're welcome!

FLAVIO: I recall when we were in Firenze you told me about an interesting experience you had with Erik Erikson. What happened?

MICHAEL: It was a long time ago, back in 1979, at the end of my postdoctoral internship. I got invited into a small, very special private study group. Erik was one of the other participants. We would meet once a month, on a certain day at 7 p.m. We took a break over the Christmas holiday, and when we resumed, Erik and I arrived at 7 p.m. – only to discover that we had all agreed to start in January at 8 p.m. The host of the meeting was busy, so he put Erik and me into the study with glasses of sherry. We chatted a bit about the time mix-up, then Erik asked what I had done over the holidays. I told him that I had gone to Italy with a girlfriend. He asked if I had gone to the Uffizi Gallery in Firenze. I had. We talked about some of the paintings, then he reminded me that, as a young man, he had been a serious art student and had spent time copying paintings in the Uffizi. We talked about Botticelli. He described, with clear recall, the way the light fell on the woman's face in a certain painting and how hard it was to capture in paint. Then he added:

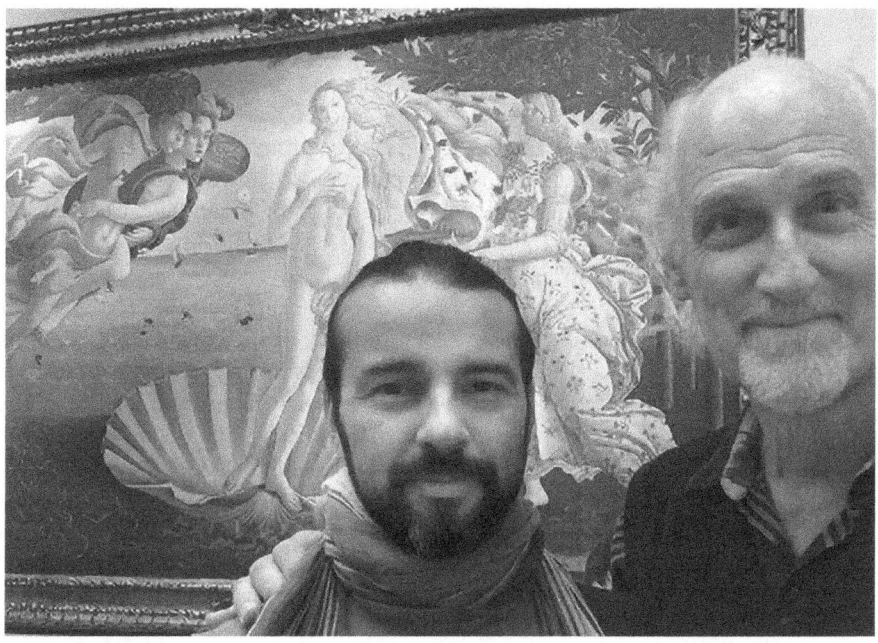

Figure 5.5 Michael and Flavio with Botticelli's *Birth of Venus*. © M.F. Hoyt. Used with permission.

"You know, it's because of art that I'm here."

"Really?"

"Yes," he said. "I was studying painting in Florence and I was spending time in the Uffizi galleries making copies and a man was there and he told me I should become a psychologist and work with children. The man was Herr Doctor Sigmund Freud. He was with his family on holiday."

FLAVIO: Fantastic!

MICHAEL: Yes. And that's why I wanted to go with you to see *The Birth of Venus*, the Botticelli painting, when we were in Florence.

FLAVIO: I remember.

MICHAEL: Number Two shout-out is for Nick Cummings. In addition to his own outstanding writing about brief therapy[44] and his professional support for psychologists and other mental-health providers (he was a President of the American Psychological Association), Nick developed large-scale healthcare systems that are venues for brief therapy. He eventually wound up building and owning a large mental healthcare company, but he started out as a chief psychologist at Kaiser Permanente, the HMO I later worked for. By the way, he was the second chief psychologist at Kaiser. The first, believe it or not, was Timothy Leary, of LSD fame! Nick said that after a year Leary left, and when the head of Kaiser hired Nick he said that if Nick screwed up, they would never hire another psychologist. Of course, Nick did a great job. Indeed, he was very proud that, years later, when they opened a new large medical center, the head of Kaiser said it was paid for by the savings in medical costs that resulted from their brief psychotherapy coverage. The head of Kaiser also told Nick that they wanted to have a psychologist, not a medical doctor, be chief of mental health services, because otherwise the strong tendency would be to address problems with medication rather than psychotherapy.

And Number Three is Jeff Zeig. Again, in addition to his own excellent contributions to psychotherapy theory and practice,[45] what Jeff has done as the Director of the Erickson Foundation and as the architect of the Evolution of Psychotherapy, Brief Therapy, Ericksonian Approaches, and Couple Therapy conferences has been truly a major gift to our field. A lot of the people I've met in our field I've met at those conferences.

We all have different influences at different stages in our development. Some involve learning specific skills, some are mentoring and personal inspiration, and some are collegial friendships. How about for you, Flavio? Who, so far, are your major influences?

FLAVIO: Well, *you* of course! [*laughing*] I mean, it's true, because you did and do a lot of work to help therapists to know about brief therapy. Having said that, I agree with all the people you mentioned – some I know more, some less. Here I should say, Giorgio Nardone gave for sure a great contribution to the evolution of strategic therapy.

MICHAEL: In what way?

FLAVIO: He took the MRI idea of attempted solutions and he created strategic protocols based on them. It's very interesting because he found that particular problems, like for example, panic attacks, have redundant attempted solutions, like avoidances or constant checking of physiological reactions. This helps to create protocols – a set of techniques, communications, and relational styles – which you can use for specific problems.[46] It's very interesting.

MICHAEL: That's good to hear.

FLAVIO: Then, in the last years, as you know, I explored BRIEF's solution-focused approach, which I love, because of its minimalism. It's a great brief therapy development. I'm finding it very useful for any kind of problem. I can say that in the last years I'm more interested in therapy based on the process than on protocols. And, last but not least, as we mentioned before, Single Session Therapy is my "North Star": How to maximize every single session.[47]

MICHAEL: Yes, indeed. I'm older, and my list could go on: Moshe Talmon and Bob Rosenbaum (my original SST buddies), of course; Carl Whitaker, the Gouldings, Steve and Insoo, Jay Haley, Don Meichenbaum[48], Michael White. And my wife, Jennifer!

FLAVIO: Yes, and my Flavia, too!

MICHAEL: We're lucky guys. There are probably other names we should cite – I apologize to those deserving folks I may not have mentioned. Simon Budman, Steven Friedman and I were co-editors of the first book I was involved with, and Alan Gurman taught me a lot as he edited versions of a couple of textbook chapters I authored.[49] Some of the other people are featured in the books I did called *Interviews with Brief Therapy Experts* (2001) and *Therapist Stories of Inspiration, Passion, and Renewal: What's Love Got to Do with It?* (2011); and in my book (2017) *Brief Therapy and Beyond*.

FLAVIO: Let's also talk about the future.

MICHAEL: Okay.

FLAVIO: What do you think will happen with brief therapy?

MICHAEL: More and more therapy will be briefer and briefer. There is a big book called *The Handbook of Psychotherapy and Behavior Change* that comes out with a new edition every few years with reviews of the latest developments. They used to have a chapter called "Brief Psychotherapies." But now most therapies *are* brief – typically six or less sessions (with one being the modal or most common length of therapy) – so they no longer have a special section called "Brief." A lot of therapy nowadays would fall under the "eclectic" rubric, and there is also a lot that's more-or-less CBT.

FLAVIO: What do you think specifically about the future for strategic therapies?

MICHAEL: I think the basic MRI mission, to promote therapy that was not long-term or psychoanalytic, has been accomplished. Now the challenge will be to see if strategic therapies can, as they say nowadays, "maintain market share." I wrote about this in an article last year,[50] and I'll be talking about this at the online conference of the Italian Scientific Society for Strategic Therapy in November 2020.

FLAVIO: What do you think the future holds for strategic therapies?

MICHAEL: I imagine five likely developments: (1) more research on methods, outcomes, and different contexts; (2) more innovative integration of different strategic approaches; (3) more awareness of cultural nuances; (4) more use of the internet for training and doing online therapy; and (5) more single-session/one-at-a-time therapies. I'm worried, however, that in-fighting among different strategic approaches and competition from CBT and from medications, as well as insurance companies favoring more individual approaches over more systemic approaches,[51] will hold back strategic therapy. I'm not sure who will be the leaders of the next generation of strategic therapists.

FLAVIO: I've noticed that when I have visited the United States, strategic therapies are not as well known or popular as they are in Europe. Why do you think that is?

MICHAEL: Several reasons. When I asked Paul Watzlawick why he thought reception for strategic/interactional therapies has been better overseas than in the United States, Paul answered: "[M]ore exposure to other languages and cultures." Americans tend to be simple and not particularly systemic or philosophic – this was true even before Trump and his stupid, destructive isolationist policies. Even someone like Giorgio Nardone, whose work is brilliant and prolific, is not much known outside of Europe. MRI's heyday was two or three decades ago, and now MRI has closed its offices in Palo Alto and exists largely as a Foundation. I was sorry they didn't sponsor the most recent Single Session Therapy Conference. It took place October 2019 in Melbourne, Australia, sponsored and hosted by The Bouverie Centre, and was excellent[52] – but I thought MRI could have benefited from the publicity. Another problem involves a relative lack of research. This is where CBT shines – they have lots of evidence from lots of researchers to support what they do. Strategic therapy also requires a lot of clever strategizing – it's difficult. I remember Steve de Shazer[53] saying strategic maneuvers were a lot of work and didn't yield any better results than finding something that clients were already doing that they could do more of. There has been a general shift toward a more collaborative, less hierarchical arrangement, more towards seeing the client as the "expert" and the "hero" in his or her own life – rather than the instrumental power being in the

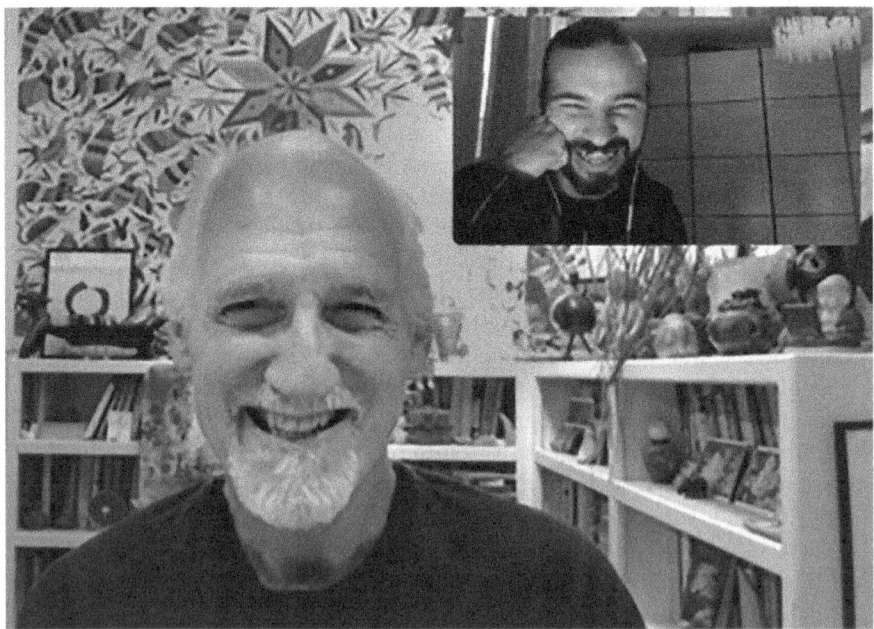

Figure 5.6 Skype screen shot, April 2020. ©M.F. Hoyt. Used with permission.

"doctor."[54] Sometimes strategic interventions seem pretty manipulative – when I was first learning about strategic therapy I thought some of the interventions sounded like they were making fun of the clients.

FLAVIO: How about Solution-Focused Brief Therapy, why do you think it has become more popular?

MICHAEL: Again, several reasons. It's usually easier and more pleasant to look for people's strengths rather than focusing on what they are doing that is not working. Insoo and Steve were much beloved, and they were both "champions" and "ambassadors" for their approach via traveling, teaching, and writing.[55] There are politics and factions within any community, but they left several leaders, organizations, and an active online international community. Evolution requires two things: environmental pressures and genetic variability, that is, emerging opportunities and the requisite skills. The SFBT move toward a more collaborative, nonhierarchical position with clients fits better with today's affirmative, respect-different-skills do-it-yourself cultural zeitgeist.

FLAVIO: It's going to be interesting to see how things go.

MICHAEL: Yes. And thanks for the opportunity to go down memory lane!

FLAVIO: Thank you for being such a wonderful mentor and friend.

Box 15. Summary of Chapter 5: A Brief History of Brief Therapy, Some Personal Influences, and Thoughts about the Future

The history of brief therapy is explored, providing an overview about several brief therapy authors and their approaches. Many anecdotes – personal or little known – help readers to better understand those authors and their thinking. Observations are also provided regarding likely brief therapy trends, as well as ideas about brief therapy training and therapist development.

Reflection Question: The authors describe how various mentors helped them at different developmental junctures. Where are you in your professional development, and where will you find the appropriate teachers/mentors?

Notes

1 M.F. Hoyt (2009). *Brief Psychotherapies: Principles and Practices*. Zeig, Tucker & Theisen. S. Freud (1937). Analysis terminable and interminable. In *Standard Edition of the Complete Psychological Works of Sigmund Freud* (J. Strachey, Ed.; Vol. 23). Hogarth Press.

2 F. Alexander & T.M. French (1946). *Psychoanalytic Therapy: Theory and Applications*. Ronald Press.

3 See N.A. Cummings & M. Sayama (1995). *Focused Psychotherapy: A Casebook of Brief, Intermittent Psychotherapy through the Life Cycle.* Brunner/Mazel.

4 M.F. Hoyt (1995). *Brief Therapy and Managed Care: Readings for Contemporary Practice.* Jossey-Bass.

5 M.F. Hoyt & S. Friedman (2000). "Dilemmas of Postmodern Practice Under Managed Care and Some Pragmatics for Increasing the Likelihood of Treatment Authorization." In M.F. Hoyt, *Some Stories Are Better Than Others* (pp. 109–117). Brunner/Mazel.

6 From p. 1, M.F. Hoyt (1995). *Op. cit.*

7 J. Haley (Ed.) (1985). *Conversations with Milton H. Erickson, M.D.* (Vols. 1–3). Triangle Press; J. Haley (1973). *Uncommon Therapy: The Psychiatric Techniques of Milton H. Erickson, M.D.* Norton. Also see J. Haley (1994). *Jay Haley on Milton H. Erickson, M.D.* Brunner/Mazel. S. de Shazer (1982). *Patterns of Brief Family Therapy.* Guilford Press. G. Bateson, D.D. Jackson, J. Haley, & J.H. Weakland (1956). "Toward a Theory of Schizophrenia". *Behavioral Science, 1,* 251–262. P. Watzlawick, J.H. Weakland, & R. Fisch (1974). *Change: Principles of Problem Formation and Problem Resolution.* Norton. R. Fisch, J.H. Weakland, & L. Segal (1982). *The Tactics of Change: Doing Therapy Briefly.* Jossey-Bass.

8 J. Haley (1973). *Uncommon Therapy. Op. cit.*; W.H. O'Hanlon (1987). *Taproots: Underlying Principles of Milton H. Erickson's Therapy and Hypnosis.* Norton; D. Short, B.A. Erickson, & R.E. Klein (2005). *Hope and Resiliency: Understanding the Psychotherapeutic Strategies of Milton H. Erickson, M.D.* Crown House Publishing; R. Battino & T.L. South (2005). *Ericksonian Approaches: A Comprehensive Manual* (2nd ed.). Crown House Publishing. Also see pp. 14–15 this volume.

9 See M. Ritterman (1983). *Using Hypnosis in Family Therapy.* Zeig, Tucker & Theisen (2nd ed., 2005).

10 See the epigraph that opens this book.

11 See G. Vitry, C. de Scorraille, & M.F. Hoyt (2021). "Redundant Attempted Solutions: 50 Years of Theory, Evolution, and New Supporting Data." *Australian and New Zealand Journal of Family Therapy, 42,* 174–187; and G. Vitry, C. de Scorraille, C. Portelli, & M.F. Hoyt (2021). "Redundant Attempted Solutions: Operative Diagnoses and Strategic Interventions to Disrupt More of the Same." *Journal of Systemic Therapies, 40*(4), 1–28.

12 W.A. Ray & S. de Shazer (Eds.) (1999). *Evolving Brief Therapies: In Honor of John H. Weakland.* Geist & Russell.

13 M.F. Hoyt (1994). "On the Importance of Keeping It Simple and Taking the Patient Seriously: A Conversation with Steve de Shazer and John Weakland." In M.F. Hoyt (Ed.), *Constructive Therapies* (pp. 11–40). Guilford Press. Reprinted in M.F. Hoyt (2001). *Interviews with Brief Therapy Experts* (pp. 1–33). Brunner-Routledge. M.F. Hoyt & I.K. Berg (1998). "Solution-Focused Couple Therapy: Helping Clients Construct Self-Fulfilling Realities." In M.F. Hoyt (Ed.), *The Handbook of Constructive Therapies* (pp. 314–340). Jossey-Bass. M.F. Hoyt (2012). "Remembering Steve de Shazer and Insoo Kim Berg." In M. Vogt, F. Wolf, P. Sundman, & H.N. Dreesen (Eds.), *Meeting Steve de Shazer and Insoo Kim Berg* [in German; pp. 73–77]. Verlag Modernes Lernen/Borgmann Publishers; reprinted in English as *Encounters with Steve de Shazer and Insoo Kim Berg* (pp. 76–80). Solutions Books, 2015.

14 In the book that resulted from that conference, Joseph Barber (1990, p. 437) wrote: "Single-session therapeutic 'cures' sometimes seem 'miraculous,' both to the therapist and to the patient, because they occur more suddenly than we expect, and because a reason for the 'cure' cannot be discerned." He noted the suggestions of Bernard Bloom (1981) to encourage single-session success, then went on (pp. 441–442):

Moshe Talmon, Michael Hoyt, and Robert Rosenbaum (1988) in their short course presentation at this Congress entitled "When the First Session is the Last: A Map for Rapid Therapeutic Change," advise us: 1. Expect change. 2. View each encounter as a whole, complete in itself. 3. Don't rush or try to be brilliant. 4. Emphasize abilities and strengths, rather than pathology. 5. Life, not therapy, is the great teacher.

See J. Barber (1990). "Miracle Cures? Therapeutic Consequences of Clinical Demonstrations." In J.K. Zeig & S.G. Gilligan (Eds.), *Brief Therapy: Myths, Methods, and Metaphors* (pp. 437–442). Brunner/Mazel; and B.L. Bloom (1981). "Focused Single-Session Therapy: Initial Development and Evaluation." In S.H. Budman (Ed.), *Forms of Brief Therapy* (pp. 167–216). Guilford Press.

15 See M. Talmon (1990). *Single–Session Therapy*. Jossey-Bass; M.F. Hoyt & M. Talmon (Eds.) (2014). *Capturing the Moment: Single-Session Therapy and Walk-In Services*. Crown House Publishing; M.F. Hoyt, M. Bobele, A. Slive, J. Young, & M. Talmon (Eds.) (2018). *Single-Session Therapy by Walk-In Or Appointment*. Routledge; M.F. Hoyt, J. Young, & P. Rycroft (Eds.) (2021). *Single Session Thinking and Practice in Global, Cultural, and Familial Contexts: Expanding Applications*. Routledge; J. Demelo (2018, July). "Bull's Eye! One-and-Done Sessions Give New Meaning to the Phrase Targeted Therapy." *O: The Oprah Magazine, 19*, 63–64, 67; M.F. Hoyt & W. Dryden (2018). "Toward the Future of Single Session Therapy: An Interview." *Journal of Systemic Therapies, 37*(1), 79–90. Also see Chapter 8 this volume.

16 J.P. Gustafson (2020). *Gaining a Second Impression in Psychotherapy: Pivoting Toward a More Accurate Understanding of the Patient*. Routledge. Also see J.P. Gustafson (1986). *The Complex Secret of Brief Psychotherapy*. Norton; J.P. Gustafson (1992). *Self-Delight in a Harsh World: The Main Stories of Individual, Marital and Family Psychotherapy*. Norton; J.P. Gustafson (1995). *The Dilemmas of Brief Psychotherapy, and Taking Care of the Patient*. Plenum Press; and J.P. Gustafson (1995). *Brief Versus Long Psychotherapy: When, Why, and How*. Jason Aronson.

17 In his Foreword to Whitaker's collected papers, Sal Minuchin (1982, p. ix) wrote:

> Like James Joyce, Whitaker creates a revolution in the grammar of life [...] Whitaker's assumption seems to be that out of his challenge to form, creative processes in individual family members as well as the family as a whole can arise ... By the end of therapy, every family member has been touched by Whitaker's distorting magic. Each member feels challenged, misunderstood, accepted, rejected, or insulted. But he has been put in contact with a less familiar part of himself.

S. Minuchin (1982). "Foreword." In J.R. Neil & D.P. Kniskern (Eds.), *From Psyche to System: The Evolving Therapy of Carl Whitaker* (pp. vii–ix). Guilford Press.

18 J.K. Zeig (Ed.) (1980). *A Teaching Seminar with Milton H. Erickson, M.D.* Brunner/Mazel.

19 John Frykman (1932–2017) was a good friend. In addition to being a skilled therapist, he was an ordained Lutheran minister and a social justice activist. See J. Frykman (2011). "Love's Got Everything to Do with It!" In M.F. Hoyt (Ed.), *Therapist Stories of Inspiration, Passion, and Renewal: What's Love Got to Do with It?* (pp. 75–86). Routledge; also M.F. Hoyt (2018). "In Memorium: Farewell, John H. Frykman, Ph.D." *The Milton H. Erickson Newsletter, 38*(1), 14.

20 For example, Carol Erickson, who was Milton's oldest daughter, told of how her father would tell her stories with complicated problems as a way of teaching her to listen, think and problem-solve at an early age. See C.E. Erickson (2011). "It Warms My Heart." In M.F. Hoyt (Ed.), *Therapist Stories of Inspiration, Passion, and Renewal: What's Love Got to Do with It?* (pp. 67–74). Routledge.

21 M.F. Hoyt (2004). "I've Always Been This Way – Thanks to Them!" In *The Present Is a Gift: Mo' Better Stories from the World of Brief Therapy* (pp. 230–244). New York: iUniverse.

22 See C.A. Whitaker & M.H. Miller (1969). "A Reevaluation of 'Psychiatric Help' When Divorce Beckons." *American Journal of Psychiatry*, 126(5), 611–618. Reprinted in J.R. Neill & D.P. Kniskern (Eds.) (1982). *From Psyche to System: The Evolving Therapy of Carl Whitaker* (pp. 196–207). Guilford Press.

23 M.F. Hoyt (2000). "A Golfer's Guide to Brief Therapy (with Footnotes for Baseball Fans)." In *Some Stories Are Better Than Others* (pp. 5–15). Brunner/Mazel. Reprinted in M.F. Hoyt (2017). *Brief Therapy and Beyond* (pp. 33–43). Routledge.

24 See M.F. Hoyt (1977). "Primal Scene and Self-Creation." *Voices: Journal of the American Academy of Psychotherapists*, 13, 24–28.

25 See Chapter 7 this volume.

26 Federico is Flavio's partner at the Italian Center for Single Session Therapy in Rome. See F. Cannistrà & F. Piccirilli (Eds.), *Terapia a Seduta Singola: Principi e Pratiche*. Giunti.

27 The paper is a chapter in J.K. Zeig & S.G. Gilligan (Eds.), *Brief Therapy: Myths, Methods, and Metaphors* (pp. 303–317). Brunner/Mazel.

28 Later Michael added: In a book of remembrances about Bob, I wrote "I don't believe in a hereafter – but some say when a star dies you can still see its light for a thousand years. Bob – Thank you. I love you." See M.F. Hoyt (1992). "Personal and Powerful." In C.L. Pelton & L. Myers-Pelton (Eds.), *Reflections of Robert L. Goulding* (pp. 179–182). Family Health Media.

29 See M.F. Hoyt (2001). "Contact, Contract, Change, Encore: A Conversation about Redecision Therapy with Bob Goulding." In M.F. Hoyt (Eds.), *Interviews with Brief Therapy Experts* (pp. 121–142). Brunner-Routledge.

30 See M. James & D. Jongeward (1973). *Born to Win: Transactional Analysis with Gestalt Experiments*. Addison-Wesley; and M. James (1985). *It's Never Too Late to Be Happy*. Addison-Wesley; E. Bader & P.T. Pearson (1988). *In Quest of the Mythical Mate: A Developmental Approach to Diagnosis and Treatment in Couples Therapy*. Brunner/Mazel.

31 R.L. Goulding (1978). "How to Catch Fish." In R.L. Goulding & M.M. Goulding (Eds.), *The Power Is in the Patient: A TA/Gestalt Approach to Psychotherapy* (pp. 1–8). TA Press.

32 M.F. Hoyt & R.L. Goulding (1989). "Resolution of a Transference-Countertransference Impasse Using Gestalt Techniques in Supervision." *Transactional Analysis Journal*, 19, 201–211. Reprinted in M.F. Hoyt (1995). *Brief Therapy and Managed Care* (pp. 237–256). Jossey-Bass. Also see M.F. Hoyt (1995). "Contact, Contract, Change, Encore: A Conversation about Redecision Therapy with Bob Goulding." *Transactional Analysis Journal*, 25(4), 300–311. Reprinted in M.F. Hoyt (2001). *Interviews with Brief Therapy Experts* (pp. 121–143). Brunner-Routledge.

33 M.F. Hoyt (1994). "On the Importance of Keeping It Simple and Taking the Patient Seriously: A Conversation with Steve de Shazer and John Weakland." *Op cit.* M.F. Hoyt (1996). "Solution Building and Language Games: A Conversation with Steve de Shazer (and Some after Words with Insoo Kim Berg)." *Op cit.* M.F. Hoyt & I.K. Berg (1998). "Solution-Focused Couple Therapy: Helping Clients Construct Self-Fulfilling Prophesies." In M.F. Hoyt (Ed.), *The Handbook of Constructive Therapies* (pp. 314–340). Jossey-Bass.

34 M.F. Hoyt & S.D. Miller (2000). "Stage-Appropriate Change-Oriented Brief Therapy Strategies." In J. Carlson & L. Sperry (Eds.), *Brief Therapy Strategies with Individuals and Couples* (pp. 289–330). Zeig, Tucker, & Theisen. Reprinted in M.F. Hoyt (2000). *Some Stories Are Better Than Others* (pp. 207–235). Brunner/Mazel.

For some of Scott's recent excellent work on Feedback Informed Treatment, see S.D. Miller, M.A. Hubble, & D. Chow (2020). *Better Results: Using Deliberate Practice to Improve Therapeutic Effectiveness.* APA Books.

35 In their 1995 book, *The Miracle Method*, Scott Miller and Insoo Berg (1995, p. 37, emphasis in original) recount the origins of the "Miracle Question," which has come to be a signature characteristic of solution-focused therapy:

> A woman called us [in 1984] for an appointment demanding that she be seen that day because it was an emergency. She began sobbing as she told the receptionist how her husband's drinking was out of control and that he had even been violent toward her. As [the client] entered the therapist's office and began to sit down, she said, "My problem is so serious that it would take a *miracle* to solve it!" [...] The therapist simply followed the client's lead, and said, "Well – suppose one happened?" Immediately, the client began to describe what she wanted to be different about the situation that was troubling her. As she described what she wanted in more detail, a smile began to creep into her face and the tone of her voice became more hopeful ... As she stood to leave the office, she told the therapist that she was feeling "much better" [...] The following week she returned and reported that she had turned that feeling into some small but significant changes in her life and her marriage.

See S.D. Miller & I.K. Berg (1995). *The Miracle Method: A Radically New Approach to Problem Drinking.* Norton.

36 See H.H. Strupp & J.L. Binder (1984). *Psychotherapy in a New Key: A Guide to Time-Limited Dynamic Psychotherapy.* Basic Books.

37 S. de Shazer (1985). *Keys to Solution in Brief Therapy.* Norton; S. de Shazer (1988). *Clues: Investigating Solutions in Brief Therapy.* Norton.

38 M.F. Hoyt (1994). "On the Importance of Keeping It Simple and Taking the Patient Seriously: A Conversation with Steve de Shazer and John Weakland." In M.F. Hoyt (Ed.), *Constructive Therapies* (pp. 11–40). Guilford Press. Reprinted in M.F. Hoyt (2001). *Interviews with Brief Therapy Experts* (pp. 1–33). Brunner-Routledge; M.F. Hoyt (1996). "Solution Building and Language Games: A Conversation with Steve de Shazer (and Some After Words with Insoo Kim Berg." In M.F. Hoyt (Ed.), *Constructive Therapies* (Vol. 2, pp. 60–86). Guilford. Reprinted in M.F. Hoyt (2001). *Interviews with Brief Therapy Experts* (pp. 158–183). Brunner-Routledge; M.F. Hoyt & I.K. Berg (1998). "Solution-Focused Couple Therapy: Helping Clients Construct Self-Fulfilling Realities." In F.M. Dattilio (Ed.), *Case Studies in Couple and Family Therapy* (pp. 203–232). Guilford. Reprinted in M.F. Hoyt (Ed.) (1998). *The Handbook of Constructive Therapies* (pp. 314–340). Jossey-Bass. Also reprinted in M.F. Hoyt (1998). *Some Stories Are Better Than Others* (pp. 143–166). Brunner/Mazel; M.F. Hoyt (2002). "Solution-Focused Couple Therapy." In A.S. Gurman & N.S. Jacobson (Eds.), *Clinical Handbook of Couple Therapy* (3rd ed., pp. 335–369). Guilford Press. Reprinted in M.F. Hoyt (2004). *The Present Is a Gift.* iUniverse. Revised version in A.S. Gurman (Ed.) (2008). *Clinical Handbook of Couple Therapy* (4th ed., pp. 259–295). Guilford. Reprinted in M.F. Hoyt (2009). *Brief Psychotherapies: Principles and Practices* (pp. 139–198). Zeig, Tucker & Theisen. Further revised version in A.S. Gurman, J.L. Lebow, & D.K. Snyder (Eds.) (2025). *Clinical Handbook of Couple Therapy* (5th ed., pp. 300–332). Guilford Press; M.F. Hoyt (2012). "Remembering Steve de Shazer and Insoo Kim Berg." In M. Vogt, F. Wolf, P. Sundman, & H.N. Dreesen (Eds.), *Meeting Steve de Shazer and Insoo Kim Berg* [in German; pp. 73–77]. Verlag Modernes Lernen/Borgmann Publishers. Reprinted in English as *Encounters with Steve de Shazer and Insoo Kim Berg* (pp. 76–80). Solutions Books, 2015.

39   See S. de Shazer (1982). *Patterns of Brief Family Therapy: An Ecosystemic Approach.* Guilford Press; also S. de Shazer (1984). "The Death of Resistance." *Family Process,* *23,* 79–93.

40   Actually, it was "MPD" and "PTSD." See p. 9 in M.F. Hoyt (1994/2001). "On the Importance of Keeping It Simple and Taking the Patient Seriously: A Conversation with Steve de Shazer and John Weakland." In M.F. Hoyt (Ed.), *Interviews with Brief Therapy Experts* (pp. 1–33). Brunner-Routledge.

41   W. Blake (1966). "Jerusalem." In D.V. Erdman (Ed.), *The Prose and Poetry of William Blake* (pp. 143–256). Doubleday. (work originally published 1804).

42   For a sample, see W.H. O'Hanlon (1987). *Taproots: Underlying Principles of Milton H. Erickson's Therapy and Hypnosis.* Norton; W.H. O'Hanlon (1999). *Do One Thing Different: And Other Uncommonly Sensible Solutions to Life's Persistent Problems.* William Morrow; W.H. O'Hanlon & A.L. Hexum (1990). *An Uncommon Casebook: The Complete Clinical Work of Milton H. Erickson, M.D.* Norton; W.H. O'Hanlon & M. Weiner-Davis (1989). *In Search of Solutions: A New Direction in Psychotherapy.* Norton; and W.H. O'Hanlon & J. Wilk (1987). *Shifting Contexts: The Generation of Effective Psychotherapy.* Guilford Press.

43   E. Erikson (1959). *Identity and the Life Cycle.* International Universities Press.

44   See, for example, N.A. Cummings & M. Sayama (1995). *Focused Psychotherapy: A Casebook of Brief, Intermittent Psychotherapy through the Life Cycle.* Brunner/Mazel. Also see N.A. Cummings (2011). "Psychotherapy's Soothsayer." In M.F. Hoyt (Ed.), *Therapist Stories of Inspiration, Passion, and Renewal* (pp. 58–66). Routledge. Dr. Cummings passed away, at age 95, on June 9, 2020.

45   See, for example, J.K. Zeig (2006). *Confluence: The Selected Papers of Jeffrey K. Zeig.* Zeig, Tucker, & Theisen; J.K. Zeig (2013). *The Induction of Hypnosis: An Ericksonian Elicitation Approach.* Milton H. Erickson Foundation Press; and J.K. Zeig (2014). *Psychoaerobics: An Experiential Method to Empower Therapist Excellence.* Milton H. Erickson Foundation Press.

46   See, for example, G. Nardone (1977). *Brief Strategic Solution-Oriented Therapy of Phobic and Obsessive Disorders.* Jason Aronson; G. Nardone & A. Salvini (2007/2018). *The Strategic Dialogue: Rendering the Diagnostic Interview a Real Therapeutic Intervention.* Routledge; G. Nardone & C. Potelli (2005). *Knowing through Changing: The Evolution of Brief Strategic Therapy.* Crown House Publishing; G. Nardone & E. Valteroni (2020). *Advanced Brief Strategic Therapy for Young People with Eating Disorders.* Routledge. For more on the theory and therapy of Redundant Attempted Solutions, also see G. Vitry, C. de Scorraille, & M.F. Hoyt (2021). "Redundant Attempted Solutions: 50 Years of Theory, Evolution, and New Supporting Data." *Australian and New Zealand Journal of Family Therapy, 42,* 174–187; and G. Vitry, C. de Scorraille, C. Portelli, & M.F. Hoyt (2021). "Redundant Attempted Solutions: Operative Diagnosis and Strategic Interventions to Disrupt More of the Same." *Journal of Systemic Therapies,* 40(4), 11–28.

47   See Chapter 8 this volume.

48   See "Cognitive-Behavioral Treatment of Posttraumatic Stress Disorder from a Narrative Constructivist Perspective: A Conversation with Donald Meichenbaum" in M.F. Hoyt (2001), *Interviews with Brief Therapy Experts* (pp. 97–120). Routledge; and "On Ethics and the Spiritualities of the Surface: A Conversation with Michael White and Gene Combs" and "Direction and Discovery: A Conversation about Power and Politics in Narrative Therapy with Michael White and Jeff Zimmerman" in M.F. Hoyt (2001, pp. 71–96 and pp. 265–293, respectively). Routledge.

49   S.H. Budman, M.F. Hoyt, & S. Friedman (Eds.) (1992). *The First Session in Brief Therapy.* Guilford Press. M.F. Hoyt (2015). "Solution-Focused Couple Therapy." In A.S. Gurman, J.L. Lebow, & D.K. Snyder (Eds.), *Clinical Handbook of Couple Therapy* (5th

ed., pp. 300–332). Guilford Press; and M.F. Hoyt (2011). "Brief Psychotherapies." In S.B. Messer & A.S. Gurman (Eds.), *Essential Psychotherpies: Theory and Practice* (pp. 387–425). Guilford Press. Dr. Gurman was also the coauthor of the influential *Theory and Practice of Brief Therapy* (Budman & Gurman, 1988; Guilford Press), and taught the first brief therapy course I took (while I was a predoctoral intern at the University of Wisconsin-Madison in 1974–1975).

50 M.F. Hoyt (2019). "Strategic Therapies: Roots and Branches." *Journal of Systemic Therapies*, 38(1), 30–43. Also see M.F. Hoyt & W. Dryden (2018). "Toward the Future of Single-Session Therapy: An Interview." *Journal of Systemic Therapies*, 37(1), 79–89 (reprinted in W. Dryden (2020). *Single-Session Therapy and Its Future: What SST Leaders Think* [pp. 31–45]. Routledge).

51 See M.F. Hoyt & A.S. Gurman (2017). "Wither Couple/Family Therapy?" In M.F. Hoyt, *Brief Therapy and Beyond* (pp. 287–293). Routledge. (A version originally appeared in *The Family Journal: Counseling and Therapy for Couples and Families*, 2012, 20(1), 13–17.)

52 Flavio and Michael were both presenters at the 3rd International Symposium. For the book that resulted from SST3, see M.F. Hoyt, J. Young, & P. Rycroft (Eds.) (2021). *Single Session Thinking and Practice in Global, Cultural, and Familial Contexts: Expanding Applications*. Routledge.

53 See M.F. Hoyt (1996/2001, pp. 159–160). "Solution Building and Language Games: A Conversation with Steve de Shazer (and Some after Words with Insoo Kim Berg)." *Op cit.*

54 See H. Anderson & H.A. Goolishian (1992). "The Client Is the Expert: A Not-Knowing Approach to Therapy." In S. McNamee & K.J. Gergen (Eds.), *Therapy as Social Construction* (pp. 25–39). Sage; B.L. Duncan, S.D. Miller, & J.A. Sparks (2004). *The Heroic Client: A Revolutionary Way to Improve Effectiveness through Client-Directed, Outcome-Informed Therapy*. Jossey-Bass. This is also part of the shift toward calling those we serve *clients* rather than *patients* (see M.F. Hoyt, 2017, *op cit.,* "'Patient' or 'Client': What's in a Name?" and "'Shrink' or 'Expander': An Issue in Forming a Therapeutic Alliance.")

55 See C.F. Visser (2013). "The Origin of the Solution-Focused Approach." *International Journal of Solution-Focused Practices*, 1(1), 10–17. Also see M. Vogt, F. Wolf, P. Sundman, & H.N. Dreesen (Eds.), *Meeting Steve de Shazer and Insoo Kim Berg* [in German; pp. 73–77]. *Op. cit.*

Part II

Extending the Conversation – Scholarly Elaborations

Single Session Therapy

A Healthful Approach to Effectively and Efficiently Solving Client Problems[1]

For almost 100 years, the dominant paradigm in clinical psychiatry, psychology, and social work has been the review of a patient's history to yield a diagnosis of disease and dysfunction, then followed by the application of professional expertise to "treat" or "cure" these putative pathologies. As Harlene Anderson has put it (in Duvall et al., 2015, p. 64), a person is placed in a category and then responded to by the clinician as "types and kinds of people with types or kinds of problems that they have read about or met before. In other words, they work from a recipe to address the person or thing in front of them." Wampold and Imel (2015) refer to this approach as the "Medical Model." The conventional emphasis has been upon the assessment of a patient's sickness and the expert treatment by the doctor.

We favor an alternative perspective, one that emphasizes individual patient/client abilities and positive future prospects. Such an approach began to be increasingly recognized with the work of Milton Erickson (1980; Haley, 1973), who emphasized *looking forward*, the *utilization of clients' own resources*, and *individualized treatment* as the preferred way to *help clients help themselves*. As Erickson wrote:

> Emphasis should be placed more upon what the patient does in the present and will do in the future than upon a mere understanding of why some long-past event occurred.
>
> (M.H. Erickson, 1954, p. 127)

and

> The fullest possible utilization of the functional capacities and abilities and the experiential and acquisitional learnings of the patient [...] should take precedence over the teaching of new ways in living which are developed from the therapist's possibly incomplete understanding of what may be right and serviceable to the individual concerned.
>
> (M.H. Erickson, 1980, p. 540)

DOI: 10.4324/9781003307709-8

and

> And I do wish that Rogerian therapists, Gestalt therapists, transactional therapists, group analysts, and all the other offspring of various theories would recognize that not one of them really recognizes that psychotherapy for person #1 is not psychotherapy for person #2.
>
> (quoted in Zeig, 1980, frontispiece)

and

> It is the patient who does the therapy. The therapist only furnishes the climate, the weather. That's all. The patient has to do all the work.
>
> (quoted in Zeig, 1980, p. 148)

Erickson (1901–1980; see pp. 14–15 this volume), being a medical doctor of his time, used the term *patient*. Most modern theorists and therapists interested in the shift toward health and strength, however, now prefer the term *client*. The former appellation tends to evoke images of pathology and dependency, whereas the latter emphasizes competence and a more egalitarian connection. Similarly, the terms used to describe the procedures (*treatment? therapy? counseling? consultation?*) convey implications about the roles of those involved, who has what powers, and what are the assumed underlying processes of change (see Hoyt, 2017, pp. 217–218).

Using skillful language to focus on and use what is healthy and good about a client has led to the publication of a number of key books, including *Uncommon Therapy: The Psychiatric Techniques of Milton H. Erickson M.D.* (Haley, 1973); the Mental Research Institute's *Change: Principles of Problem Formation and Problem Resolution* (Watzlawick et al., 1974) and *The Tactics of Change: Doing Therapy Briefly* (Fisch et al., 1982); de Shazer's *Keys to Solution in Brief Therapy* (1985) and *Clues: Investigating Solutions in Brief Therapy* (1988); O'Hanlon and Weiner-Davis's (1989) *In Search of Solutions: A New Direction in Psychotherapy*; and White and Epston's *Narrative Means to Therapeutic Ends* (1990). While they draw from different theoretical and technical approaches, they all have in common the overarching idea and attitude that, with some facilitation, clients have the competence and motivation to make changes and solve their own problems. Their emphasis is on health, not sickness. As Seligman and Csikszentmihalyi, advocates for "positive psychology," put it (2000, p. 7):

> Our message is to remind our field that psychology is not just the study of pathology, weakness, and damage; it is also the study of strength and

Table 6.1 Solution-Building Vocabulary

In	Out	In	Out
Respect	Judge	Forward	Backward
Empower	Fix	Future	Past
Nurture	Control	Collaborate	Manipulate
Facilitate	Treat	Options	Conflicts
Augment	Reduce	Partner	Expert
Invite	Insist	Horizontal	Hierarchical
Appreciate	Diagnose	Possibility	Limitation
Hope	Fear	Growth	Cure
Latent	Missing	Access	Defense
Assets	Defects	Utilize	Resist
Strength	Weakness	Create	Repair
Health	Pathology	Exception	Rule
Not Yet	Never	Difference	Sameness
Expand	Shrink	Solution	Problem

From Hoyt (1994, p. 4) ©1994 M.F. Hoyt. Used by permission.

virtue. Treatment is not just fixing what is broken; it is nurturing what is best.

And yet, as de Shazer pointed out (in Hoyt, 1994, p. 20), conventional psychotherapy has been a mental *illness* industry, rather than a mental *health* industry. Nardone and Salvini (2007, p. 104) similarly commented:

> Often, in contrast to what one might think, it is the psychologist and psychiatrist who are resistant to this paradigmatic leap; their cognitive resistances are functional to keep up their identity in line with the social expectancies of the role they hold.

In 1994, the fundamental shift toward health was described by Hoyt as "competency-based future-oriented therapy." In a series of edited volumes, Hoyt (1994, 1996a, 1998) used the general term "constructive therapies" to denote positive, health-oriented therapy approaches. Table 6.1 highlights some of these shifts:

In some later publications, Hoyt (e.g., 2015, 2017) also described a "Context of Competence" [see Box 8 from Chapter 3, pp. 66–67 this volume] in which effective therapy is conceptualized at occurring at the intersection of Alliance, Goals, and Resources: therapeutic change happens when, facilitated via the therapeutic alliance, the client's resources (capacities, health) are used to achieve the client's goals.

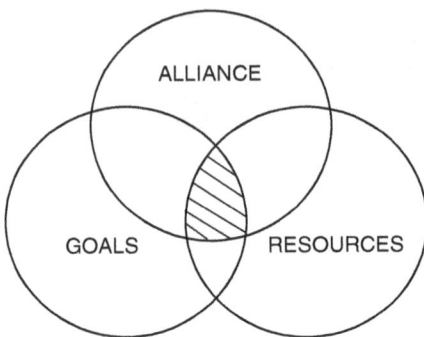

Figure 6.1 Context of competence. (From Hoyt, 2015. © M.F. Hoyt 2015. Used with permission.)

Single-Session Therapy

Intercurrent with these developments, Moshe Talmon, Robert Rosenbaum, and Hoyt were exploring the possibilities of single-session therapy (SST), what might be accomplished in one meeting. Their initial research, involving a series of 58 consecutive outpatients, resulted in the book *Single-Session Therapy: Maximizing the Effect of the First (and Often Only) Therapeutic Encounter* (Talmon, 1990; also see Talmon, 1993). They reported the following results:

- Over half of the patients (58.6%) elected to complete their therapy in one session even when more sessions were available;
- More than 88% reported significant improvement in their original "presenting complaint," and more than 65% also reported "ripple" improvements in related areas of functioning; and
- While not experimentally assigned to one-session or longer, on follow-up there was no difference in satisfaction and outcome scores between those who chose to stop after one visit (SST) versus those who continued for more sessions.

As Rosenbaum (1994) wrote, a single-session approach is a forum for "intrinsic integration," drawing upon whatever the client and therapist can bring to help solve the client's problems. "The ultimate goal of therapy is its conclusion" (Loriedo & Vella, 1992, p. 125). Therapy should not be "long" or "short" – it should be "as few sessions as possible, not even one more than is necessary" (de Shazer, 1991, p. ix). Not only does "every session count" (Preston et al., 1995) – when you're only going to meet once, every moment counts![2]

An SST "mindset" includes the three interrelated key themes of (1) expectation, the belief that one session could be enough; (2) time, the belief that change can occur in the moment; and (3) empowerment, the belief that clients have the capacity to alter their thoughts, emotions, and behaviors to bring about beneficial changes (Talmon & Hoyt, 2014). A series of SST general principles have been offered (Talmon, 1990; Rosenbaum et al., 1990; Hoyt & Talmon, 2014, p. 4) that reflect these themes:

- Expect change.
- View each encounter as a whole, complete in itself.
- Do not rush or try to be brilliant.
- Emphasize abilities and strengths rather than pathology.
- Life, not therapy, is the great teacher.
- More is not necessarily better. Often less is more. In any case, better is indeed better.
- Big problems do not always require big solutions. Be pragmatic.
- The essence of therapy is more about helping clients to help themselves than about the therapist's need to be needed.
- Most clients have limited resources (time and money) and these should be preserved and respected.
- Terminate in a way that allows the client to realize useful implications.

Using an integrated variety of competence-oriented approaches, the frequent effectiveness of SST has now been repeatedly demonstrated in a wide variety of situations, involving clients and clinicians from different countries and continents, addressing different problems and using different theories and methods (see Slive & Bobele, 2011; Cannistrà & Piccirilli, 2018; Dryden, 2018; Hoyt & Talmon, 2014, 2018; Hoyt et al., 2018). Readers are encouraged to consult those publications and others in the bibliography.

SST and the Health-Based View

As Young (2018) has written, SST is a planned one-session "delivery system." This is, in our opinion, a very positively disruptive/reframing way to look at psychotherapy and its capacity to help people. As Slive and Bobele (2018) explained, people normally attend common-life "walk-in" services: restaurants, cinemas, banks, hairstylists, etc. These are all examples of services in which a client simply walks in and expects that he or she will find what they need in one session. Even many medical services work like this. The main reason why psychotherapy is instead mostly viewed as a more-than-one-session service – and the reason why therapists themselves act like this – is because of our theories. As Fisch (1994, p. 126) wrote, therapy "was brief until the advent of psychoanalytic concepts and practices near the turn of this century." We think that this is a provocative – and stimulating – idea. While it is obvious that psychoanalysis has made great contributions to the psychotherapy field, we also know that "how we look determines what we see, and what we see influences what we do" (Hoyt, 2009). That is, if we think that a person with a problem needs many sessions (many years?) to solve it, it probably will be so. Is this absolutely wrong? No. But it could be a wrong absolutism.

Observing that the reason why a large number of people decide to attend for "only" one session is "because it helped me" (Talmon, 1990; Westmacott & Hunsley, 2010; Simon et al., 2012), the single-session therapist approaches each session with the belief that one session could be all that the client will need. Hoyt (2011, p. xii) and Bobele and Slive (2014) refer to this as "one-at-a-time." Young (2018) notes that this is another chance to deliver the therapy. Plus, it implies that the therapist thinks that the client has the resources to help herself. After all, as Cannistrà (2019) wrote, the therapist could be useful in many ways, for example, by helping the client:

- To solve her problem;
- To elaborate strategies that she can apply on her own;
- To start or consolidate the change process;
- To conceive and answer questions during crises or emergencies;
- To talk about something important for her. This doesn't mean that the therapist must provide answers "as an expert." Rather, the client may think: "Let's see if an expert can help me to figure out something."

In his Foreword to Talmon's *Single Session Therapy*, Jerome Frank (1990) noted that the idea of clients being able to make changes in one session of therapy violates or challenges a lot of assumptions that have guided conventional therapists: the belief that you have to gradually form an alliance, the belief that you have to gradually uncover the underlying schemas or conflicts, and the belief that you then have to gradually work your way through or there will be too much resistance. When things happen in one session, it's an interesting challenge for theoreticians and researchers, because it can't be a gradual working-through process; something shifted more quickly.

We don't want to deny the suffering of clients nor neglect the existence and utility of therapies that need many sessions to be helpful. But just as Paul Watzlawick (1990a, 1990b) would help clients solve problems by advising that they act "as-if" they could solve (or already had solved) the problem, we believe that embracing a health-based view is better than assuming that health is a difficult destination to reach. Every psychotherapy works on a series of assumptions, as if those assumptions are "true." Assumptions can be the basis for "self-fulfilling prophecies." To work as if one session could be enough, with the chance to do other sessions if needed, seems to us a useful, economical, and respectful assumption. People's self-healing capacities are one of the most important therapeutic factors in therapy (Asay & Lambert, 1999; Bohart & Tallman, 1999).

Two SST Case Examples

While each case is conceived idiographically, keeping with the idea that it is the unique resources of clients that can make a healthy difference, we offer these two examples as typical.

Clinical Example 1: A Case of Obsessive Thoughts

Paolo came to the office complaining of "obsessive thoughts." Ten years prior he had started to suffer from intrusive images of him hurting his wife and children with knives or in some other way. In that first episode, he took some medication for six months and the problem vanished for eight years, after which it returned. Not wanting to resume medications (partially because of side-effects), he then read a book about brief therapy and tried to use a paradoxical intervention (thinking voluntarily of the images instead of fighting them), and again the images vanished. But, in the last six months, the images came again, this time also with obsessive worries about his job, his family's health, money, the future, and so on. "Every day I lose myself in distressing thoughts, imagining the worst scenarios for me and my family."

I (FC) listened very carefully to the story, giving Paolo feedback about his successes (e.g., "So, you're telling me you lived eight years without the problem? How did you do that?" and "What do you mean when you say that you followed the suggestions in the book? What did you do?"). My intention was to help to focus Paolo's attention on an important thing: he had already been successful. At that point, I complimented him for his successes with the obsessive images and I said that they seemed to me very good strategies. Then I asked him if he thought that he could use the paradoxical intervention again, maybe with a little adjustment. He said, "Yes" and I suggested that he use the technique five minutes every day, for three weeks: "It's just a more systematic way to use what you did before" (see Nardone & Watzlawick, 1993). After that, I asked him if in the last months he had also found a good strategy for the worries. He told me that he had: when the worries would come, he would try to distract himself, sometime saying to himself, "They are all bullshit." I laughed and said that it seemed to me to be a good way, and asked how well it worked. It does work, he said, so I suggested he use it again, more systematically. Paolo agreed and smiled. At this point I said that it seemed to me that we had two good strategies for the problems he had brought and I asked if he wanted to discuss something else and if he thought he needed a second session. He said "No" to both, so we agree to have a telephone call in three weeks, to see how things were going. At that time, Paolo reported that the problem was no longer present. He said that he had experimented with the paradoxical intervention and in a few days the obsession that he had for six months had vanished and the worries, connected to real-life problems, had become "normal worries a man has to confront."[3]

Comment. Emphasizing "what works" and having the SST mindset that emphasizes positive expectations, time, and empowerment, the client's past success with paradoxical intervention had been identified and reinforced (de Shazer, quoted in Hoyt, 1996b, p. 68, advised: "Once you know what works do more of it"). Various brief therapy logics (Cannistrà, 2019; also see Chapter 7, this volume), including *Create Awareness* (helping the client to be more aware of something – in this case of his resources and successful strategies) and *Increase to Reduce* (do more of something to provoke a paradoxical effect – in this case using the paradoxical intervention), were applied.

Clinical Example 2: A Case of Couple Therapy

George and Mary arrived complaining of communication problems and unhappiness. They had been married for seven years and had two children. They each said that they still loved the other, but they felt they were no longer "as happy as before." I (MFH) complimented them for wanting to make things better and asked them what would be a small step in the right direction. They mentioned good times they had had in the past – dates, adventures, and time to be alone together. Following their lead, I asked about how they had met and got lots of details about fun and pleasure. They began to recall seeing one another as sources of light, not darkness; they laughed and began to rekindle hope. We talked about ways they could take turns and better listen to one another. We also acknowledged some of the difficulties of having two small children at home (I told a brief normalizing story about my wife and I when our son was a small child), and we talked about ways they could schedule some time to be together without the kids. To heighten their receptivity, I strategically asked: "If things don't get better, they could get worse, right?" They agreed they didn't want that. Drawing from narrative therapy (White & Epston, 1990), I explored with them their answers to the question of how they could keep parenting and fatigue from destructively getting between them. At a moment when it looked like they might revert into demoralizing problem talk[4], I interjected the solution-focused Miracle Question (de Shazer, 1988, p. 5):

> Hey, suppose tonight while you're sleeping, a miracle happens and the problems that brought you here are resolved! Tomorrow, when you wake up, how will you notice that the miracle had occurred? What would be the first signs? And then?

By the end of the meeting they were feeling encouraged, had skills and plans ready, and did not think another appointment would be necessary but agreed to call back as needed.

Comment: Consistent with a SST mindset, a variety of techniques were integrated to promote client empowerment, problem-solving and a positive future orientation. The therapist directly asked the couple what would be for them a small step to the right direction, then amplified it by asking successful examples from their past. Perceptive readers may note that the question "How will you notice when things are better?" contains the Ericksonian supposition/suggestion that good things would happen.

In both cases, the therapists didn't assume that there was "something wrong needing to be fixed." They could have, of course, but they preferred to focus their attention – and that of the clients – on healthy behaviors, previous successful solutions and strategies proposed by the clients that fit well with the clients' personal characteristics. This empowered clients' self-confidence, promoted positive perspectives, and built on what had worked – and would work – for the clients.

In every given moment we can add complexity to the therapeutic process, for example, by trying to understand the problem using personality models, attachment theories, meta-cognition analyses, and so on. But to us it seems that starting from the simplest point – adding complexity only later, if necessary – can be the better, easier, and briefer way to help clients.

Conclusion

SST promotes patient self-care and can have a beneficial and significant impact on the finances of large healthcare delivery systems. As Hoyt et al. (2018, p. 15) have noted, however, "There remains a serious need for increased funding for all mental-health and other social services" and "SST is not a panacea, but when included as part of a range of services [...] SSTs can meet immediate needs and also help make more resources available for clients truly needing them" (Hoyt et al., 2018, p. 374).

Abundant evidence (see Hoyt & Talmon, 2014; Hoyt et al., 2018, 2021) clearly demonstrates that SST is, de facto, the most common length of therapy. While all problems cannot be successfully addressed in SST (or other brief or long-term therapy), many can – especially when the therapist is oriented toward the possibility of effective one-session-at-a-time therapy and is on the lookout for whatever client strengths can be utilized to help resolve the presenting problem. The future (see DeMelo, 2018; Hoyt & Dryden, 2018) of SST is bright and healthy.

Notes

1 Appeared originally in *Italian Journal of Mental Health* (*Rivista Sperimentale di Freniatria*), 2019, *143*(1), 73–85 [in English and Italian]. Used with permission.

2 Michael later added (from Hoyt, 2017, p. 11):

> I am reminded of an experience I had long ago [1978] when I visited the Short-Term Therapy Seminar at the renowned Tavistock Clinic in London (Malan, 1963, 1976a, 1976b). Cases were presented and I was asked to comment, which I did with some trepidation. We got into a discussion about length of treatment. I indicated that at the clinic where I was then working, we generally saw patients for twelve sessions, a number that followed Mann's (1973) time-limited psychotherapy model and allowed a good research design (Horowitz et al., 1984). "Here at the Tavistock we allow trainees thirty-five to forty sessions. It allows for wasting time and making mistakes," I was told. "Well, in America we're more efficient," I responded. "We find that we can waste time and make mistakes in twelve sessions!"

3 While preparing this book, Flavio did another telephone follow-up, two years after the single session. Paolo reported that he once had a little relapse during a moment of great stress, but that the problem was now completely solved and the obsessions

were gone. He commented, "Now it's okay. Sometimes the thoughts come and I watch them and let them flow away."

4 See George et al. (1990) and Furman and Ahola (1992) for discussions of the distinction between *problem talk* and *solution talk*.

References

Asay, T.P., & Lambert, M.J. (1999). The empirical case for the common factors in therapy: Quantitative findings. In M.A. Hubble, B.L. Duncan, & S.D. Miller (Eds.), *The Heart and Soul of Change: What Works in Therapy* (pp. 23–55). American Psychological Association.

Bobele, M., & Slive, A. (2014). One session at a time: When you have a whole hour. In M.F. Hoyt & M. Talmon (Eds.), *Capturing the Moment: Single Session Therapy and Walk-In Services* (pp. 95–119). Crown House Publishing.

Bohart, A.C., & Tallman, K. (1999). *How Clients Make Therapy Work: The Process of Active Self-Healing*. American Psychological Association.

Cannistrà, F. (2019). A violent life: Using brief therapy "logics" to facilitate change. In M.F. Hoyt & M. Bobele (Eds.), *Creative Therapy in Challenging Situations: Unusual Interventions to Help Clients* (pp. 47–57). Routledge.

Cannistrà, F., & Piccirilli, F. (2018). *Terapia a Seduta Singola: Principi e Pratiche*. Giunti.

DeMelo, J. (2018). Bull's-eye! One-and-done sessions give new meaning to the phrase *targeted therapy*. *O: The Oprah Magazine*, July, 63–64, 67.

de Shazer, S. (1985). *Keys to Solution in Brief Therapy*. Norton.

de Shazer, S. (1988). *Clues: Investigating Solutions in Brief Therapy*. Norton.

de Shazer, S. (1991). Foreword. In Y.M. Dolan (Ed.), *Resolving Sexual Abuse: Solution-Focused Therapy and Ericksonian Hypnosis for Adult Survivors* (pp. ix–x). Norton.

Dryden, W. (2018). *Single-Session Therapy: 100 Key Points and Techniques*. Routledge.

Duvall, J., Carleton, D., & Tremblay, C. (2016). Reengaging history with Harlene Anderson: Nosie Rosie *goes!* Part I. *Journal of Systemic Therapies, 34*(4), 61–79.

Erickson, M.H. (1954). Special techniques of brief psychotherapy. *Journal of Clinical and Experimental Hypnosis, 2*, 109–129.

Erickson, M.H. (1980). *Collected Papers* (Vols. 1–4; E.L. Rossi, Ed.). Irvington.

Fisch, R. (1994). Basic elements in the brief therapies. In M.F. Hoyt (Ed.), *Constructive Therapies* (pp. 126–139). Guilford Press.

Fisch, R., Weakland, J.H., & Segal, L. (1982). *The Tactics of Change. Doing Therapy Briefly*. Jossey-Bass.

Frank, J.D. (1990). Foreword. In M. Talmon (Ed.), *Single-Session Therapy* (pp. xi–xiii). Jossey-Bass.

Furman, B., & Ahola, T. (1992). *Solution Talk: Hosting Therapeutic Conversations*. Norton.

George, E., Iveson, C., & Ratner, H. (1990). *Problem to Solution: Brief Therapy with Individuals and Families*. Brief Therapy Press.

Haley, J. (1973). *Uncommon Therapy: The Psychiatric Techniques of Milton H. Erickson, M.D.* Norton.

Horowitz, M.J., Marmar, C., Krupnick, J., Wilner, N., Kaltreider, N., & Wallerstein, R. (1984). *Personality Styles and Brief Psychotherapy*. Basic Books.

Hoyt, M.F. (Ed.) (1994). *Constructive Therapies*. Guilford Press.

Hoyt, M.F. (Ed.) (1996a). *Constructive Therapies 2*. Guilford Press.

Hoyt, M.F. (1996b). Solution building and language games: A conversation with Steve de Shazer. In M.F. Hoyt (Ed.), *Constructive Therapies 2* (pp. 60–86). Guilford Press.

Hoyt, M.F. (Ed.) (1998). *The Handbook of Constructive Therapies.* Jossey-Bass.

Hoyt, M.F. (2009). *Brief Psychotherapies: Principles and Practices.* Zeig, Tucker, & Theisen.

Hoyt, M.F. (2011). Foreword. In A. Slive, & M. Bobele (Eds.), *When One Hour Is All You Have: Effective Therapy for Walk-In Clients* (pp. ix–xv). Zeig, Tucker, & Theisen.

Hoyt, M.F. (2015). Solution-focused couple therapy. In A.S Gurman, J.L. Lebow, & D.K. Snyder (Eds.), *Clinical Handbook of Couple Therapy* (5th ed., pp. 300–332). Guilford Press.

Hoyt, M.F. (2017). *Brief Therapy and Beyond: Stories, Language, Love, Hope, and Time.* Routledge.

Hoyt, M.F., Bobele, M., Slive, A., Young, J., & Talmon, M. (Eds.) (2018). *Single-Session Therapy by Walk-In or Appointment: Administrative, Clinical, and Supervisory Aspects of One-at-a-Time Services.* Routledge.

Hoyt, M.F., & Dryden, W. (2018). Toward the future of single-session therapy: An interview. *Journal of Systemic Therapies, 37*(1), 79–89.

Hoyt, M.F., & Talmon, M. (Eds.) (2014). *Capturing the Moment: Single-Session Therapy and Walk-In Services.* Crown House Publishing.

Hoyt, M.F., & Talmon, M. (2018). *Prefazione.* In F. Cannistrà & F. Piccirilli (Eds.), *Terapia Seduta Singola: Principi e Pratiche* (pp. ix–xiv). Giunti.

Hoyt, M.F., J. Young, J., & Rycroft, P. (Eds.) (2021). *Single Session Thinking and Practice in Global, Cultural, and Familial Contexts: Expanding Applications.* Routledge.

Loriedo, C., & Vella, G. (1992). *Paradox and the Family.* Brunner/Mazel.

Malan, D.H. (1963). *A Study of Brief Psychotherapy.* Tavistock Publications.

Malan, D.H. (1976a). *The Frontier of Brief Psychotherapy.* Plenum.

Malan, D.H. (1976b). *Toward the Validation of Dynamic Psychotherapy.* Plenum.

Mann, J. (1973). *Time-Limited Psychotherapy.* Harvard University Press.

Nardone, G., & Salvini, A. (2007). *The Strategic Dialogue: Rendering the Diagnostic Interview a Real Therapeutic Intervention.* Karnac. (reissued 2018 by Routledge)

Nardone, G., & Watzlawick, P. (1993). *The Art of Change.* Jossey-Bass.

O'Hanlon, W.H., & Weiner-Davis, M. (1989). *In Search of Solutions: A New Direction in Psychotherapy.* Norton.

Preston, J., Varzos, N., & Liebert, D. (1995). *Every Session Counts: Making the Most of Your Brief Therapy.* Impact Publishers.

Rosenbaum, R. (1994). Single-session psychotherapies: Intrinsic integration? *Journal of Psychotherapy Integration, 6,* 107–118.

Rosenbaum, R., Hoyt, M.F., & Talmon, M. (1990). The challenge of single-session therapies: Creating pivotal moments. In R.A. Wells, & V.J. Giannetti (Eds.), *Handbook of the Brief Psychotherapies* (pp. 165–89). Plenum Press.

Seligmann, M.E.P., & Csikszenmihalyi, M. (2000). Positive psychology: An introduction. *American Psychologist, 55,* 5–14.

Simon, G.E., Imel, Z.E., Ludman, E.J., & Steinfeld, B.J. (2012). Is dropout after a first psychotherapy visit always a bad outcome? *Psychiatric Services, 63*(7), 705–707.

Slive, A., & Bobele, M. (Eds.) (2011). *When One Hour Is All You Have: Effective Therapy for Walk-In Clients.* Zeig, Tucker, & Theisen.

Slive, A., & Bobele, M. (2018). The three top reasons why walk-in/single-sessions make perfect sense. In M.F. Hoyt, M. Bobele, A. Slive, J. Young, & M. Talmon

(Eds.), *Single-Session Therapy by Walk-In Or Appointment: Administrative, Clinical, and Supervisory Aspects of One-at-a-Time Services* (pp. 27–39). Routledge.

Talmon, M. (1990). *Single-Session Therapy: Maximizing the Effect of the First (and Often Only) Therapeutic Encounter.* Jossey-Bass.

Talmon, M. (1993). *Single Session Solutions: A Guide to Practical, Effective, and Affordable Therapy.* Addison-Wesley.

Talmon, M., & Hoyt, M.F. (2014). Moments are forever: SST and walk-in services now and in the future. In M.F. Hoyt, & M. Talmon (Eds.), *Capturing the Moment: Single-Session Therapy and Walk-In Services* (pp. 463–485). Crown House Publishing.

Wampold, B.E., & Imel, Z.E. (2015). *The Great Psychotherapy Debate: The Research Evidence for What Works in Psychotherapy* (2nd ed.). Routledge.

Watzlawick, P. (1990a). *Psychotherapy "As If."* Presentation at Second Evolution of Psychotherapy Congress, December 12.

Watzlawick, P. (1990b). Therapy is what you want it to be. In J.K. Zeig, & S.G. Gilligan (Eds.), *Brief Therapy: Myths, Methods, and Metaphors* (pp. 55–61). Brunner/Mazel.

Watzlawick, P., Weakland, J.H., & Fisch, R. (1974). *Change: Principles of Problem Formation and Problem Resolution.* Norton.

Westmacott, R., & Hunsley, J. (2010). Reasons for terminating psychotherapy: A general population study. *Journal of Clinical Psychology, 66*(9), 965–77.

White, M., & Epston, D. (1990). *Narrative Means to Therapeutic Ends.* Norton.

Young, J. (2018). Single-session therapy: The misunderstood gift that keeps on giving. In M.F. Hoyt, M. Bobele, A. Slive, J. Young, & M. Talmon (Eds.), *Single-Session Therapy by Walk-In Or Appointment* (pp. 40–58). Routledge.

Zeig, J.K. (Ed.) (1980). *A Teaching Seminar with Milton H Erickson, M.D.* Brunner/Mazel.

Chapter 7

The 9 Logics Beneath Brief Therapy Interventions

A Framework to Help Therapists Achieve Their Purpose[1]

Brief therapies use different kinds of operations, interventions, tasks, and techniques. Discussing strategic therapy, Jay Haley (1963; 1973, p. 1) wrote that "Therapy can be called strategic if the clinician initiates what happens during therapy and designs a particular approach for each problem," and went on (1973, p. 17) to note that strategic therapy isn't "a particular approach or theory, but a name for the types of therapy where the therapist takes responsibility for directly influencing people." Haley, of course, was inspired by his years of study with the well-known psychiatrist Milton Erickson (Haley, 1985). In *Uncommon Therapy*, Haley (1973) described many different interventions by Erickson, whose work influenced many different kinds of brief therapies. Whether we talk about the development of strategic therapies (e.g., Watzlawick et al., 1974; Fisch et al., 1982; Nardone & Watzlawick, 1993), solution-focused therapies (e.g., de Shazer, 1988; O'Hanlon & Weiner-Davis; 1988; Berg & Miller, 1992), or other types of brief therapies (see Hoyt, 1994, 1996, 1998, 2000, 2001, 2017), we can recognize the centrality of active interventions. As Levy and Shelton (1990, p. 145, italics in original) said, tasks are not seen "as an adjunct, even a critical adjunct to brief psychotherapy. Rather, we see them as *the basis for action in brief psychotherapy*. If therapy is to be effective in a short period of time, the therapist *must* encourage the efficient conduct of the client's therapeutic activities – both in and outside of the therapy session."

But what is the purpose of a technique? Why does a therapist choose to give a particular task rather than another? Or, as Steve de Shazer (1985, p. 3) said: "How did you decide to use that particular intervention?" A few pages later, de Shazer (1985, p. 8) also noted: "The rules behind the interventions were unclear. The only thing certain was that the various cases involved specific behavioral concerns with specific behavioral interventions with a specific goal in mind."

But does that lead to the idea that *every* different technique or task or intervention produces a different effect? Is it possible that for every single therapy technique – even for just the ones typically associated with different brief therapies – there is a different logic, a different result that the therapist wants to achieve?

DOI: 10.4324/9781003307709-9

We think not, and that was the start of this study, which seeks to help the therapist to know better what could be the best intervention(s) to achieve a particular purpose with a specific person in a specific session.

Why "Logics"

First, it is necessary to explain what is meant by the term *logic*. We choose to use a broad meaning of the term, as described by the Italian dictionary (Treccani, 2019, 3c): "The reason that underlies a particular behavior and that justifies it."[2] It seems to us that the term *logic* can include meanings like reason, purpose, intention, desired result/effect, and goal. The basic idea is that when a therapist does (or assigns) a specific intervention or uses a specific tactic, it is because he or she means to achieve a specific effect. The therapist has the idea that the intervention will act in a certain way, hoping that following a logic will bring the desired result. Regarding terminology: "logic" is preferable to "strategy" because "strategy" implies a more complex plan, made up of a series of maneuvers and tactics. As Rampin (2004, p. 80) says: "the whole course of the therapy corresponds [to the strategy], that is the succession of the sessions."

Some Contact Points: Similarities and Differences with Other Studies

The idea of underlying logics, even with different names, behind the choice of one technique or another is not new in brief therapy. Different kinds of techniques can be included in the same logic. Using the terms of mathematics, we could say that different elements (techniques) can be part of the same set (logic).[3]

In *Keys to Solution in Brief Therapy*, Steve de Shazer (1985, p. 10) commented that many people would ask "How does the brief therapist know what to do, and how to do it?" and "Where did *that* intervention come from?" Later in the same book, de Shazer noted (pp. 59–60) that an intervention is not "like a specific key designed to fit a specific lock," but rather, invoking the concept of *fit*, suggested that "It is only that the intervention needs to fit in the way a skeleton key is designed to be used in a variety of locks, without considering the particulars of the type or shape of lock." A lock (problem) can be opened by different keys (interventions). We add that many keys can belong to the same bunch, or they are the same kind of key: double-sided, four-sided, transponder, dimple, paracentric. Those bunches correspond to the different logics.

In *Clues: Investigating Solutions in Brief Therapy*, de Shazer (1988) provided some general guidelines for designing tasks – such as making an exception to the rule, or changing the location, or who is involved, or adding a new element to the pattern, or increasing its duration, and so on. In the work discussed below, such interventions are part of a logic we call *small changes*, because they all aim to ask the client to introduce a small difference in his or her behavior or to do a small step.

Dan Short, Betty Alice Erickson and Roxanna Erickson-Klein (2005; also see Short, 2021), in the book *Hope and Resiliency: Understanding the Psychotherapeutic Strategies of Milton H. Erickson, M.D.*, describe six core strategies underlying Milton Erickson's techniques:

1 *Distraction*. Shifting the client's attention away from self-defeating experiences to ones that promote health and success.
2 *Partitioning*. Breaking down of negative association by dividing a boundless problematic reality into smaller, more easily assimilated parts.
3 *Progression*. Building on a series of small gains, creating increased hope for continued accomplishments.
4 *Suggestion*. Collecting and guiding the patient's expenditure of energy [...] to elicit a response that somehow exceeds the bounds of what the patient believed to be possible prior to therapy.
5 *Reorientation*. Providing the patient with a new perspective, a view of the situation that reduces the amount of subjective distress.
6 *Utilization*. Attending to the goodness of the patient's mind and body, using their energy, preferences, point of view, skills and potentials.

Some of the work of Short et al. is similar to the "logics" we describe below. For example, *distraction*, *partitioning*, and *progression* are close to the logics *shift the focus* and *small changes* and both are intended to bring about a specific result that the therapist wants to achieve in order to solve the problem. But, on the other hand, *suggestion*, *reorientation*, and *utilization* are not specific results the therapists want to achieve. Those are techniques or interventions they use *to produce* an effect. As we will see, following Cannistrà (2018a, 2019), we have identified nine logics that help the therapist to identify *prior* to intervention what therapeutic effect they want to produce, facilitating the process of choosing a specific technique that they think to be the best or the more suitable for that client in that situation.

Again, similar to our *small changes* logic is Zeig's (1999, p. 137) description of a way to proceed in therapy (a "logic," we could say) in which

> the therapist has in mind a tailored main intervention. This could be a symptom prescription, ordeal, or anecdote. Rather than moving directly to the main course, however, the therapist [...] proceeds in small steps toward the main intervention, which is succeeded by a period of follow-through. This procedure has been named SIFT. The therapist moves in Small steps, Intervenes, and then Follows Through.

DeJong and Berg (1997, pp. 120–133) advised that, if the clients view the problem as existing outside of themselves but are able to identify random exceptions, the therapist could ask them, every night before they go to bed, to predict whether or not the next day *something* will or will not happen; at the end of the next day, the clients must write down if the prediction came true. In the present work, this prescription could follow the logic *creating awareness*, if the therapist would have the client pay attention to something that he or she thinks is already happening; or *create from nothing*, if the therapist wants to "push" the client to start to perceive a brand-new reality. The same technique could be used for different purposes, so the logic of intervention will be different.

In his book *Taproots: Underlying Principles of Milton Erickson's Therapy and Hypnosis*, Bill O'Hanlon (1987, pp. 36–37) suggested some ways to intervene on a symptom, for example, changing the frequency, rate, duration, time of the day, location, intensity, sequence, etc. The "way" can be "the intervention" but not the effect. That is, in our vision, the therapist chooses to change frequency, rate, duration, etc., *because* he or she wants to achieve a specific goal, to produce a specific effect: he or she is following a specific logic. In particular, all of O'Hanlon's aforementioned interventions could be included under the same logic, which we call *small changes* (the therapist asks the client to do some "little things," some "small changes," to produce a particular effect the therapist believes will lead to the final result of an improvement), whereas when O'Hanlon (1987, pp. 43–48) talks about "linking the occurrence of the symptom/pattern to another negative/undesired pattern" we included it in the logic of *create aversion*.

In the writings of Palo Alto's Brief Therapy Center (Watzlawick et al., 1974; Fisch et al., 1982; Fisch & Schlanger, 1999) there is frequent use of *paradoxical interventions* (see also Weeks & L'Abate, 1982; Loriedo & Vella, 1992), a category of interventions which in our study is part of those interventions that the therapist does with the idea (the logic of) *increase to reduce* a behavior, a feeling, a symptom, etc.

In their book *The Logic of Therapeutic Change*, Giorgio Nardone and Elisa Balbi (2008/2018) identified three kinds of logics underlying problems and their solutions. They call them *the logics of ambivalence*, saying that they are three kinds of not-ordinary logics:

- *Logic of paradox*: "two contradictory messages are present at the same time within a communicational structure" (p. 62, Italian edition);
- *Logic of contradiction*: when the client says/does something and then does/says the opposite;
- *Logic of belief*: "the logical criterion that refers to all that we can structure as something in which we believe, which does not necessarily correspond to a thought or a cognition" (p. 69, Italian edition).

Nardone and Balbi (2008/2018, p. 71, Italian edition) say: "Accordingly, we can develop operative techniques for therapeutic changes based on these three logics, which in order to operate, must of course be tailored to the problem in order to be corrected." For those authors, every problem could be looked at from one of these three logics, and the solution (the therapeutic intervention, and in particular the tactic that the therapist chooses to use) seems to fit with the same logic of the problem. In the present work, however, we don't conceptualize the logic of the problem. We assume that the therapist thinks what is the effect he or she wants to produce or what is needed to help the client: this is the logic that will guide their intervention. Furthermore, differently from Nardone and Balbi, we haven't hypothesized some underlying logic of the problems, but we have started to analyze techniques to derive the possible logics that the therapist follows when he chooses to use them.

Again Nardone (2003), in a brief dissertation on the ancient arts of Greek and Chinese strategy and persuasion, identified 13 "essential stratagems," which are "formulas applicable to many different situations [...] Each stratagem does not represent a simple recipe to copy, but a principle to be learned to build 'ad hoc' interventions" (p. 35). This is very similar to the idea behind the concept of "logic": if you know the right logic (the "principle," in Nardone's words), you can choose/build the right intervention. We also find that some stratagems correspond almost exactly with our proposed logics: Nardone's *to sail the sea without the knowledge of the sky* corresponds to our *shift the focus*; Nardone's *if you want to straighten something, learn first how to distort it more* is similar to our *create aversion*; Nardone's *extinguish the fire by adding wood* is basically the same of our *increase to reduce*; and we adopted the same name of the stratagem *create from nothing*.

Methodology

As described by Cannistrà (2018a, 2019), numerous books and articles were initially reviewed, all written by therapists working with MRI's strategic therapy (Watzlawick et al., 1974; Fisch et al., 1982); Brief Strategic Therapy (Nardone & Watzlawick, 1993); Solution-Focused Brief Therapy (SFBT) (de Shazer et al., 2007); plus many techniques most directly derived from Milton Erickson's works (Haley, 1973, 1975; Erickson et al., 1976; Erickson & Rossi, 1980, 1981). Other brief therapies (e.g., see Cannistrà & Piccirilli, 2018; Hoyt & Talmon, 2014; Hoyt et al., 2018, 2021; Zeig & Munion, 1999) were then considered that were more or less influenced by those approaches or authors. At the beginning, 77 techniques were examined (13 have since been added, the number now being 90).

For every single technique, the reason was considered why the therapist used that particular technique, wondering what was the effect they hoped to produce. Basing on that, the underlying logic was determined.

For example, in Nardone et al. (1999/2005) the authors talk about a prescription, the *aesthetic report card*, in which the therapist asks an anorexic girl to have a relaxing bath and then, in front of a mirror for ten minutes, she has to give herself a rating for every single part of her body. The declared effect is "to provoke in the girl an emotional experience" (p. 80 in the Italian edition) that brings her to new perceptions of herself. This is the effect the therapist wants to produce. The therapist could do that in many ways, but decided to use that particular intervention: everyday, for ten minutes, she has to give herself a rating. This could follow at least two logics: one is that the therapist would bring the girl to see that she isn't "fat" or "ugly" (a logic we call *creating awareness*); another is that he wants to ask her to do something she never did before: take care of her body, feeling new sensations and having new perspectives (what we call *create from nothing*).

At first, we wrote down all the plausible logics for every technique. A technique could be under more than one logic. In this phase we just wanted to see how many logics, how many reasons we could find for why a therapist does an intervention. After having analyzed 77 techniques, we identified 9 different logics and were able to always put a technique in at least one of them.

At that point, we started to reduce the complexity, limiting every single technique to the one or two logics we thought were most representative of it. For every technique, we identified a "main logic" (the most likely for that intervention) and a secondary logic, if there was one.

It should be noted that, working from a radical constructivist (Watzlawick, 1984; von Glasersfeld, 1995) and social constructionist (Gergen, 1991) viewpoint, we are fully aware that, as von Foerster (1984) said, there isn't an observation without an observer, which means that our view is not "THE reality," it is just a point of view. Others might see more logics, less logics, and/or different logics, or put some techniques under other logics – or just see anything but logics! As Watzlawick said (in Hoyt, 2001, p. 155), "the task of scientific research is the development of methods and techniques that are useful for a specific purpose, but will certainly be replaced by more effective approaches within a few years." We think about this system as a "complexity reducer," that is, as Watzlawick (in Poerksen, 2001, p. 184) said, "an incursion that does not destroy high complexity but only reduces it to useful and manageable proportions."

Results: Nine Logics

The result of this initial work is the identification of nine logics. We'll identify some techniques under each logic, but it's important to understand that a technique can be included in different logics: it is the way the technique is used that makes the difference. Moreover, our study began analyzing formalized techniques (i.e., techniques that usually have specific procedures – sometimes even specific words to say, or even specific names that identify them), but to enlarge our examples we'll present both formal techniques and more generic interventions that help to illustrate every single logic. We do not mean to suggest that a cited author was necessarily the inventor or originator of a particular approach.

Direct Block of Actions. The main purpose of this logic is to *directly* block an attempted dysfunctional solution (Watzlawick et al., 1974), or more than one, or in general a particular behavior that perpetuates the problem. "Direct" means explicitly asking the patient to stop doing a certain thing: checking, asking for help, asking for advice, looking for an answer (thinking about it, asking others or consulting different media), talking about the problem, helping someone, and giving suggestions. Many interventions are designed to block the attempted dysfunctional solutions (especially in MRI-influenced therapies) or to block a certain behavior. Those that fall under this logic, however, have the purpose of blocking them through the direct request for a behavior to be ceased. Other techniques might block the behavior being considered problematic without the block being required directly (Erickson et al., 1976; Erickson & Rossi, 1980; Nardone & Watzlawick, 1993).

Some examples of *direct block of attempted solutions* include:

- Hypochondriacal behavior is maintained by clients going continuously to doctors and specialists to ascertain their problem; in Brief Strategic Therapy (Nardone, 1996) clients are therefore directed to stop any medical examinations.
- The ritualistic behavior of certain obsessions and compulsions often involves the intervention of others, who thus maintain the problem; the others must therefore be warned to stop helping (Pietrabissa et al., 2016).
- In so-called "obsessive doubt" the person continues to look for an answer that leads to another question; therefore, the client is asked to stop giving answers to inhibit the questions. The same applies to others when they respond to the client's requests for answers.
- In many problems, talking about the problem itself is not a functional solution, rather it keeps alive the problem and concerns about it; clients therefore are asked not to talk about the problem (Nardone & Watzlawick, 1993, named this *conjury of silence*).
- The therapist can also ask others to stop certain behaviors in order to help the client. "For instance, the MRI group might help the depressed person's family stop aggravating the situation by stopping the family's efforts 'to cheer him up.' [...] In turn, this 'stopping of the cure' can help the depressed person become less depressed or even help him stop being depressed" (de Shazer, 1982, pp. 28–29).

Create Aversion. This logic includes those techniques aimed at creating in the client an aversion towards something, such as to a behavior, or to a form of interaction or relationship, etc., which leads to spontaneously stopping that behavior or preventing it from being implemented. The therapist doesn't directly ask the client to stop doing something but can use some interventions to push the client to do that.

Some examples of *create aversion* include:

- The technique *fear of help* (Nardone, 1996), in which during the session it is noted to the anxious client that all the times when he asks for help to perform a task that he feels is too difficult, he receives the implicit confirmation that "You are not capable" – with the purpose of creating their aversion to this request for help. The therapist can also use this logic in a homework assignment, e.g., by asking the client to think about it five minutes every day.
- Another example is the technique of *poor me*, conceived by Leonardi and Grassi (2012), in which the client is asked to make a list of bad things he does and then repeat them every morning while looking in the mirror. Often people quickly begin to dislike those things and stop complaining. The therapist can also use *poor me* as an in-session exercise.
- An *ordeal task* could be used as a particular variant of this logic. Talking about how to treat insomnia, Martiny (1989, p. 130) says that "a task assignment was used to make it more desirable to sleep than carry out the tasks." The purpose of assigning such an "ordeal" (Haley, 1985) is to make it more inconvenient to carry out the symptomatic behavior than to let it go. For someone with insomnia, assigning a pointless or boring task might make sleep a desirable escape; a couple might have to contribute money to a political opponent if they don't go out together on a date to spend it (Hoyt, 2019a).
- Another example is the so-called *how worse* technique (Fisch et al., 1982; Nardone & Watzlawick, 1993), in which the therapist asks the client to think about all the things she can do to *make worse* (not improve) a certain situation/problem/symptom/etc. In this way, the technique is used to create an aversion to the behaviors/patterns related to them, so that the client spontaneously stops them. Ruess' (1997) "Nightmare Question" ("Imagine when you wake up things are worse!") is an example; Hoyt (2019a) also reports directing a man who was flirting with divorce to visit the local pancake house on Sunday morning to see all the unhappy fathers and kids having breakfast before the kids ended their weekend visitations "since that may be where you're heading anyway."
- *Reframing* interventions could be used to create aversion. They could be used in a more-or-less direct and/or sophisticated way, as in this example: A depressed man described himself as a "workaholic." He admitted that he pushed himself mercilessly, never took more than two or three days of vacation and then only rarely, and so on. The therapist was able to reframe his depression as a beneficial force, by explaining to the client that his depression was forcing him to stay away from work and take it easy at home – a luxury, if not a necessity, that he would never purposely allow himself. The client found this explanation a profound and useful "interpretation" and stopped trying to force himself to feel more

lively and outgoing. Predictably, his depression diminished (Fisch et al., 1982, p. 135).

Create Awareness. This series of interventions are meant to help the client become aware himself or herself of something that generally could be either a positive/good/useful resource or strength or a problematic behavior/habit/ attitude. Interventions intended to *activate the client's strength* (Soo-Hoo, 2018, 2019) fit here. As Soo-Hoo has noted, while Duncan et al. (2009) found 30% of treatment outcome variance could be attributed to "relationship factors," they also found that 40% was related to "client factors" such as the client's strengths, resources, and motivation. If calling awareness to problematic behaviors or attitudes, the therapist doesn't mean necessarily to create antipathy for something with the idea to stop it – not immediately, anyway. This logic could also be used to make someone aware of others' (good/bad) behaviors. The therapist can create awareness of this in more-or-less direct ways. She can directly indicate positive resources or dysfunctional behaviors; or she can use a maieutic (Socratic mode of inquiry) approach (Cannistrà, 2018b); or she can use metaphors, aphorisms, or stories (Lankton & Lankton, 1983).

> Even if what is brought by the client may be initially considered dysfunctional, utilization grants the therapist the ability to build upon client actions and to channel clients' experiences into a more resourceful outcome [...] Utilization helps therapists avoid clashes with clients over change.
>
> (Leslie, 2019, pp. 80–81)

Once you know the logic, you can adapt it in various ways. Some examples of *creating awareness* include:

- Calling attention to and emphasizing the client's skills and abilities. This might be done when a therapist elicits information about a client's hobbies and interests (as part of *utilization* – Erickson, 1959; Battino & South, 2005; Short et al., 2005); when an SFBT therapist pursues solution-talk (e.g., Furman & Ahola, 1992; Walter & Peller, 1992) or when the therapist asks, *a lá* Insoo Kim Berg, "Wow – how did you do that?!"; or when MRI therapists Karin Schlanger and Esther Krohner (2019) declare, "Our clients *are* able and strong."
- The *search for confirmation* technique, which asks a person who strongly believes that others talk badly about her or plot against her to actively seek confirmation of this by observing the faces of the people to find traces of expression that betray their intentions. As seen in a case reported by Cannistrà (2019), this technique often yields exactly the opposite effect since the person actively seeking confirmation instead of staying isolated "within his mind" doesn't find confirmation, and this makes him aware that maybe he is wrong.

- The aforementioned *how worse* technique, used to create aversion, could also be used to creating awareness. This is an example of how the technique follows the therapist's logic. If one wants simply to make the client aware about some (his or others') bad behaviors, without the idea to create aversion or antipathy but just to make the client more conscious of them, he can use this technique.

- Another example is the technique of *measuring the limits* (Nardone, 1996), in which a client with a specific phobia for a given animal is asked to measure how close he manages to get to it: by doing this the person begins to realize that his fear is not so big and that the phobic object is not so scary; Andreas (2014; Andreas & Andreas, 1989) reports a similar NLP-based technique in which the subject imaginally approaches a feared object.[4]

- *Compliments*, often used in SFBT, are used also to create awareness about specific things. For example, they

    > highlight the actions the [client] has already undertaken to reach a solution [...] frame the responsibility and credit for change as the [client's] accomplishment. In a supportive climate, cheerleading and compliments combine to give [clients] a sense of self-efficacy, empowerment, and motivation.
    >
    > (Burg & Mayhall, 2002, p. 83)

- The *search for exceptions* (de Shazer et al., 1986), another feature of SFBT, is a series of questions and/or between-session prescriptions "designed to find out what happens when the complaint does not happen and how the [client] gets this exception to happen" (p. 215) that can be used to help the client to be more aware of "what works" (i.e., what the client and/or his environment are doing that is useful). In fact,

    > not only can this discussion lead to some models for intervention design and solution, but it implicitly lets the client know that the therapist believes that they not only can do but already are doing things that are good for them.

- In Batesonian (1972) terms, the exceptions at least implicitly provide the client with "news of a difference" between what works and what does not work.

Evoke New Resources. This logic includes techniques that are designed to create or amplify resources, skills and abilities in the client, introducing changes (small or large) in their perceptions and behaviors, often with the idea of starting something to do or look at something in a new way. They appear to be creating something where there was nothing. The therapist can direct the client to do that or, again, she can try to elicit it in a more indirect way.

Some examples of *create from nothing* include:

- The *Miracle Question* technique (de Shazer, 1988), which asks the client to imagine a future without the problem – or rather, the future when this problem will be no more – and to implement the behaviors that the client imagines would lead to such a future. Sometimes you can ask the client directly to do something *as if* the miracle has happened, while other times you can just ask the client to *notice* new, different, or simply "better" things that will be happening (Ratner et al., 2012).
- *Scaling questions* (Berg & de Shazer, 1993) can function similarly. A way to use them is when the therapist asks the client to notice, between sessions, all the things (generally connoted as strengths and resources) that will tell him or her that he or she is on a higher step of the scale than the one on which they are currently positioned. Or the therapist can also ask the client *to do* something as if they are on that step.
- Many *as if* interventions (Watzlawick, 1987) fall under this logic. The therapist asks the client to do/imagine/speak about something *as if* a particular condition is present (e.g., acting as if the client deserves the love of others; acting as if she feels more self-confidence; speaking as if he's an excellent lecturer; etc.), with the idea to produce new behavior and/or new meanings.
- Different *reframing* (see Watzlawick et al., 1974, p. 95; Paoli, 2014; Hoyt, 2017, pp. 242–245) interventions may involve these techniques when they are used to show to the client a new perspective, a new reality, within which to begin to use different behaviors. The therapist follows this logic when she wants the client to reach or build new meanings. This can be done also with the *creating awareness* logic, of course, and probably with several other interventions (and logics) – after all, creating new meaning is one of the purposes of psychotherapy. But when the therapist is following other logics, to create a new meaning is not the final purpose, the last (or a subsequent) goal to be reached. Instead, when the therapist is using *create from nothing* logic, doing these kinds of interventions, she wants specifically to create a new meaning in that moment or with that intervention.
- Watzlawick (1997; see also Nardone & Salvini, 2018) talked about a *planned casual event* wherein the therapist plans a strategy, suggests a task, or asks some questions in an apparently casual way to produce a discovery effect from which the client realizes or does something new.

Increase to Reduce. Many brief therapy techniques and interventions are designed to ask the client to do more of something (such as a particular behavior) with the precise intent to eventually reduce the behavior; that is the general purpose of *paradoxical interventions*, in which "the behavior the client wants to change or eliminate is prescribed or encouraged by the therapist" (Weeks & L'Abate, 1982, p. 6). The idea of the therapist is to "dissolve one thing by increasing it to the breaking point. To feed to reduce. To raise to inhibit" (Nardone, 2003, p. 71), sometimes with the idea "of making voluntary the spontaneous reactions we want to inhibit," other times with the idea to "show something to hide it" (Nardone, 2003, p. 75), e.g., when the therapist asks the client to make his embarrassment explicit instead of trying to hide it. For a case example of someone being asked to increase obsessive checking as a way to ultimately reduce it, see Hoyt and Cannistrà (2019; Chapter 6 this volume). The general aim is to ask a client to increase the frequency, duration or intensity of a behavior or a symptom, with the therapeutically intended opposite effect of reducing it.

Some other examples of *increase to reduce* include:

- The *worst fantasy* technique (Haley, 1985; Nardone & Watzlawick, 1993), in which the client with panic attacks is asked to try to increase the feelings of anxiety to paroxysmal levels, resulting in contrast a reduction of them.
- The *check-up* technique (Nardone, 1996), in which a client who thinks that she has one or more terrible diseases, for which she always tends to control herself and listen to her body, is asked to do three times a day for 15 minutes a careful examination of her body, from head to foot. The result often is that the client returns with a strong reduction of the controlling behavior and symptomatology.
- This logic also can be used during the dialogue with the client. For example, Weakland et al. (1974, p. 161) said:

  [W]e almost routinely stress "going slow" to our patients at the outset of treatment and, later, by greeting a patient's report of improvement with a worried look and the statement, "I think things are moving a bit too fast." We also do the same thing more implicitly, by our emphasis on minimal goals, or by pointing out possible disadvantages of improvement to patients. "You would like to do much better at work, but are you prepared to handle the problem of envy by your colleagues?" Such warnings paradoxically promote rapid improvement, apparently by reducing any anxiety about change and increasing the patient's desire to get on with things to counteract the therapist's apparent overcautiousness.

- Rosen (1982, p. 33) wrote that "Haley has also pointed out that major features of Ericksonian therapy include 'encouraging resistance,' 'providing a worse alternative,' [...] 'amplifying a deviation,' and 'prescribing the symptom.'"

Small Changes (or Small Violations). This logic includes those techniques aimed at solving a problem by implementing small, both incremental and decremental, changes. This is a very typical intervention that we can find in many brief therapy approaches. Milton Erickson, for example, said, "I would want to improve it in a very minor way. As soon as I got the slightest minor change in it, the way would be open for a larger change" (quoted in Haley, 1973, p. 291). Thus, Haley (1982, p. 23) also wrote: "The small change invariably led to the larger one. As Erickson put it, if you want a large change you should ask for a small one." At MRI, Weakland et al. (1974, p. 150) similarly set forth:

> We contend generally that change can be effected most easily if the goal of change is reasonably small and clearly stated. Once the patient has experienced a small but definitive change in the seemingly monolithic nature of the problem most real to him, the experience leads to further, self-induced changes in this, and often also, in other areas of his life.

At Milwaukee's Brief Family Therapy Center, de Shazer's (1988) Miracle Question would ask: "What will be the *first small signs* that this miracle has happened and that the problem is solved?"

The reasons to follow this logic can be several: the issue is composed of different steps, to be addressed one at a time; or too fast or too large results may scare the client or otherwise put him or her into trouble; or generally when the therapist must proceed slowly for any reason. The techniques ask clients to do something that does not require excessive effort, thus producing changes gradually.

Some examples of *small changes (or small violations)* include:

- The technique of *small violations* (Nardone & Portelli, 2005, 2013), used, for example, with OCD, consists in asking the client to make voluntary small violations, small differences in their rituals or compulsive behavior, in order to subvert them and to produce a gradual change.
- Asking an insecure client, who finds it difficult to present himself for fear of receiving a refusal, to put himself everyday in the situation to receive from someone a "No" of modest size. This is very effective to "immunize" him.
- The *interval technique* (Nardone et al., 1999/2005), which asks a person who vomits after eating to interpose an interval (say, of one hour) between the binge and vomit. This produces a gradual violation of the vomiting ritual.
- In treating depression, Yapko (1997, 2016) highlights the value of asking the client to do small steps, breaking complex activities into small behaviors.

Strengthen the Relationship. Although some interventions may have "collateral" effects on specific or general aspects of the therapeutic alliance, this is the only one of the nine logics that is not intended to *directly* produce a therapeutic result.[5] However, it is essential in all those cases in which without work on the relationship the therapy could be stuck or the client at risk to drop out – for example, the client would not do what is prescribed, or she or he disagrees with the reasons she or he is in therapy, or with the role assumed by the therapist, etc. The intention of the therapist could be to enhance the client's trust or hope about therapy, its effectiveness, or the therapist's skills. It could be also to create a good climate, to reassure the client and to communicate that therapy is a "safe place," e.g., assuring an adolescent that everything they say will stay in the room. The therapeutic relationship and alliance are the most important factors to determine the effectiveness of therapy, and they are composed of different parts (Norcross, 2011).

Some examples of *strengthen the relationship* include:

- The *Dear Doctor* technique (Nardone et al., 1999/2005), which asks the client to write, every night, a letter to the therapist, speaking of himself, his problems, his day and all that is in his mind. Although there are many writing techniques (e.g. "diaries"), what differentiates this is the recipient and the subject of the letters. Nardone et al. explicitly use them to improve the alliance with clients having eating disorders.
- One of the main effects of *speaking the client's language* is exactly to improve the relationship between the client and the therapist (Watzlawick, 1978; Shaw & Magnuson, 2006).
- Assuming a *one-down position* (Watzlawick et al., 1967) could be done intentionally to enhance the relationship (Fisch et al., 1982; see Hoyt, 2019b). MRI's John Weakland was a real master in doing this. In fact, "By putting himself down, Weakland disarms highly critical, suspicious, and opinionated people and puts them more at ease" (Green, 1995, p. 232).
- *Compliments*, often used in SFBT, have many functions. One of them can be to reinforce the alliance between therapist and client (Bannink, 2010).

Shift the Focus. Many techniques can be designed to shift the client's attention; in general, the client can focus on a task not realizing he is doing something else. However, this category includes techniques that, by asking the client to do a certain thing, prevent the client ("distraction") from making another response that would continue the problem. The therapist can use this technique when she thinks that directly asking the client to do something is too much for him. Many indirect interventions are in this logic, but it is important to understand that this is not the category of all the indirect interventions.

Some examples of *shift the focus* include:

- The aforementioned *planned casual event* (Watzlawick, 1997) can be used when a therapist asks the client to do something with the idea to achieve another result, focusing on the finger to reach the moon, or "to sail the sea without the knowledge of the sky" (Nardone, 2003).
- When Erickson (Rosen, 1982) asked a client who had fear to cross the street to send him a postcard, he shifted the focus of the client to a task he

could accomplish (sending a postcard) and thus allowed him, in this way, to do something he had great difficulty doing (crossing the street).

- Nardone and Rampin (2015) posit that premature ejaculation is often maintained by the client's effort to delay the ejaculation, and it is therefore necessary to block this (delaying) behavior. To do so, they found it better not to ask directly (which would reflect a *direct block of attempted solution* logic) but to ask the client to quickly ejaculate so as to focus on a second round of intercourse. In this case, the attempted solution is blocked but not with a direct request: the client's attention is rather moved to another task, which, indirectly, leads to blocking the attempted dysfunctional solution.

- The *logbook technique* (see Nardone & Watzlawick, 1993), in which the person in an acute state of anxiety is asked to fill out a diary at that exact moment: this shifts the focus from the monitoring of physiological conditions (accelerated heartbeat, tremors, sweating, etc.), the monitoring of which only exacerbates these conditions, on to a completely different task (filling in the diary), thus making it possible for the physiological conditions to recover independently.

- The indirection of a police officer asking for a cup of coffee as a way of separating a domestically disputing couple (Everstine & Everstine, 1983); or the charming Japanese folktale (retold by de Shazer, 1991) of a villager who, unable to warn his neighbors of an impending tidal wave, set their hillside terraces on fire so that they rushed up the mountain to battle the flames and thus inadvertently were saved from drowning.

Express and Process. This last category includes all those techniques that aim to express and/or process a particular lived experience at the time when the problem is precisely maintained by the continuous and excessive retention of such experience (e.g., feelings of anger or unexpressed pain) and its failure to process. The techniques in this category lead to the emergence of different feelings when there usually has been a retaining of them, or more or less incomplete processing. Budman and Gurman (1988, p. 89), speaking about the use of techniques used for loss that, in our opinion, can be grouped in this logic, say that "it may give the patient the opportunity to try to give meaning to and to gain mastery over loss." The intention of the therapist is not to "interpret" something but to help the client to face and let out some contents, feelings, thoughts, and actions. The main idea is also not just to make the client more aware about the contents (*creating awareness* logic). In MRI's view, this could be a way to stop an unsuccessful attempted solution: the client could hold some feelings and the therapist asks the client to express them.

Some examples of *express and process* include:

- *Anger letters* (Cagnoni & Milanese, 2009), in which the person with impulsive outbursts is asked to write letters daily addressed to the object of his anger, with the result that the anger is reduced and the impulsive behaviors are too;

- A similar technique is the *criminal novel* (Cagnoni & Milanese, 2009), often used for Post-Traumatic Stress Disorder, in which the client is asked to rewrite the trauma scene;
- Budman and Gurman (1988, p. 88) suggest *regrieving*,

  a powerfully emotional "reliving" of the loss, such as looking at photographs of the deceased, visiting significant locations such as gravesites or the site of a trauma, or using hypnosis to encourage time regression to the point of the trauma or before it.

- Another example is the *memory gallery* (Nardone, 1998; also see Gershman & Thompson, 2019), in which a person who has suffered the loss of a loved one and avoids a confrontation with his experiences is asked to review a gallery of paintings that represent memories related to the object of loss in order to facilitate the process of elaboration.

Each technique can serve multiple logics, although they normally fall under no more than two categories, one of which is primary. We need to remember that a technique is but an instrument obeying the logic of intervention: once the latter is identified, the therapist can derive and produce techniques.

Applications

We have started to train students and colleagues with this method. While waiting for further input and feedback on the utility of conceptualizing nine logics, we have already experienced three ways in which they can be useful.

- *When a technique doesn't work.* When a technique or an intervention doesn't work, the therapist will often try another technique, thinking that that will fit better. Unfortunately, sometimes it doesn't. Why? Often because the therapist is using a different technique but the same logic. In other words, the therapist changed the element but is still in the same set.

Having in mind the nine logics, the therapist can more easily see if it is better to change the guiding logic. Steve de Shazer said (1985, p. 13), "If it works, don't fix it"; but he also said, "If it doesn't work, then don't do it again, do something different." The point here is that you must do "a difference that makes a difference" (Bateson, 1972, p. 465) which, in our consideration, is moving from one logic to another. The nine logics give a framework for thinking, a reference with which the therapist can reflect on what is the best intervention in that moment, for that problem, with that person. In our experience, it is very hard to consider more than two logics before you find the right one for that problem at that time with that person.

- *When the client doesn't do the task (or they "resist").* Sometimes, the client doesn't do the task or homework that was assigned in the previous session, or we try an intervention in session and the client "resists." When this happens, sometimes the therapist persists with that same task or intervention, sure that it's "the right thing to do" (maybe because "the books" – or the supervisors – say so). Other times, the therapist may try a different technique, but the new one still doesn't work. Sometimes even when the logic is correct, the specific technique/intervention used isn't. It's possible that, for whatever reason, that particular intervention simply doesn't fit for that person, even if the logic, the goal, is correct. Recognizing the right logic, we can easily find a different technique within the same set.
- *When the therapist doesn't know what to do.* It is not only younger therapists who find themselves in situations in which they don't know what the right intervention is, or what could be a useful technique to use for that client, in that moment. Often, in these cases, clinicians simply "try" something that they *feel* may be right, or that seems similar to something they read about or heard about in their training. This is somewhat akin to rolling dice and hoping that a winning number comes up. Instead, using the nine logic frame, the therapist can easily build or select a new technique, one fitting with the person/problem she meets, by thinking of the right logic to use.

Conclusion

The concept of "logics" can be useful to help therapists to improve their work with clients. Considering the logic beneath an intervention is a way:

- To avoid being stuck and not knowing what to do;
- To be more creative, inventing new techniques;
- To fit a particular client's needs, adapting/creating the right technique for the person.

Different techniques could serve the same purpose. The same technique could also be used to serve a different logic or purpose. When a technique does not seem to be working, it can be helpful to ask: "What am I trying to accomplish?" (This can also be useful to ask in supervision.) You may need a different method to achieve your purpose, or you may need a different purpose. What is the underlying logic of your intervention?

"Logics" are just a framework, not an absolute: we're sure that different eyes will see different scenarios – maybe different logics, maybe more, maybe less. "How you look determines what you see, and what you see influences what you do – around and around" (Hoyt, 2009). We hope our point of view had produced a useful tool and a new starting point.

Notes

1 This is a slightly expanded and updated version of the article that appeared originally in *Journal of Systemic Therapies*, 2020, *39*(1), 19–34. Used by agreement.
2 The *English Oxford Dictionary* (retrieved online 28 January 2019) similarly defines *logic*: "a system or set of principles underlying the arrangements of elements in a computer or electronic device so as to perform a specified task." As we discuss below, Nardone and Balbi (2008/2018) have also used the term *logics*.
3 Of course, this also implies that the same element/technique can be part of different sets/logics, both by its nature (as a cat can be part of both "felines" and "pets") and depending on the use that is made of it (as a knife can be part of both "cutlery" and "weapons").
4 Again, the therapist could use these techniques with another purpose to gradually expose the client to the phobic object. In this case, the techniques will follow under the *small changes* logic.
5 A therapist could consider that for a specific client it would be directly therapeutic to strength the relationship with the therapist himself, perhaps to provide "support" or bolster the client's confidence. Generally speaking, however, the therapeutic relationship is the vehicle, not the destination.

References

Andreas, S. (2014). SST with NLP: Rapid transformations using content-free instructions. In M.F. Hoyt & M. Talmon (Eds.), *Capturing the Moment: Single-Session Therapy and Walk-In Services* (pp. 277–298). Crown House Publishing.

Andreas, C., & Andreas, S. (1989). *Heart of the Mind: Engaging Your Inner Power to Change with NLP*. Real People press.

Bannink, F. (2010). *Handbook of Solution-Focused Conflict Management*. Hogrefe.

Bateson, G. (1972). *Steps to an Ecology of Mind: Collected Essays in Anthropology, Psychiatry, Evolution, and Epistemology*. University of Chicago Press.

Battino, R., & South, T.L. (2005). *Ericksonian Approaches: A Comprehensive Manual* (2nd ed.). Crown House Publishing.

Berg, I.K., & de Shazer, S. (1993). Making numbers talk: Language in therapy. In S. Friedman (Ed.), *The New Language of Change* (pp. 5–24). Guilford Press.

Berg, I.K., & Miller, S. (1992). *Working with the Problem Drinker: A Solution-Focused Approach*. Norton.

Budman, S.H., & Gurman, A.S. (1988). *Theory and Practice of Brief Therapy*. Guilford Press.

Burg, J.E., & Mayhall, J.L. (2002). Techniques and interventions of solution-focused A advising. *NACADA Journal, 22*(2), 79–85.

Cagnoni, F., & Milanese, R. (2009). *Cambiare il Passato. Superare le Esperienze Traumatiche con la Terapia Strategica*. Ponte alle Grazie.

Cannistrà, F. (2018a, December 6) *The 9 Logics Beneath Brief Therapy Interventions*. Short course presented at Brief Therapy Conference sponsored by Milton H. Erickson Foundation, Burlingame, CA.

Cannistrà, F. (2018b). Il metodo dell'Italian Center for Single Session Therapy. In F. Cannistrà, & F. Piccirilli (Eds.), *Terapia a Seduta Singola. Principi e Pratiche* (pp. 89–118). Giunti.

Cannistrà, F. (2019). A violent life: Using brief therapy "logics" to facilitate change. In M.F. Hoyt & M. Bobele (Eds.), *Creative Therapy in Challenging Situations: Unusual Interventions to Help Clients*. Routledge.

Cannistrà, F., & Piccirilli, F. (Eds.) (2018). *Terapia a Seduta Singola. Principi e Pratiche.* Giunti.

DeJong, P., & Berg, I.K. (1997). *Interviewing for Solutions.* Brooke/Cole.

de Shazer, S. (1982). *Patterns of Brief Family Therapy.* Guilford Press.

de Shazer, S. (1985). *Keys to Solution in Brief Therapy.* Norton.

de Shazer, S. (1988). *Clues: Investigating Solutions in Brief Therapy.* Norton.

de Shazer, S. (1991). *Putting Difference to Work.* Norton

de Shazer, S., Berg, I.K., Lipchik, E., Nunnally, E., Molnar, A., Gingerich, W., & Weiner-Davis, M. (1986). Brief therapy: Focused solution development. *Family Process, 25*(2), 207–221.

de Shazer, S., Dolan, Y., Korman, H., Trepper, T., McCollum, E., & Berg, I.K. (Eds.) (2007). *More than Miracles: The State of the Art of Solution-Focused Brief Therapy.* Routledge.

Duncan, B.L., Miller, S.D., Wampold, B., & Hubble, M. (2009). *The Heart and Soul of Change: Delivering What Works in Therapy* (2nd ed.). APA Books.

Erickson, M.H. (1959). Further clinical techniques of hypnosis: Utilization techniques. *American Journal of Clinical Hypnosis, 2*(1), 3–21.

Erickson, M.H., & Rossi, E.L. (1980). Indirect forms of suggestion. In E.L. Rossi (Ed.), *The Collected Papers of Milton H. Erickson on Hypnosis: Vol. 1. The Nature of Hypnosis and Suggestion* (pp. 452–477). Irvington.

Erickson, M.H., & Rossi, E.L (1981). *Experiencing Hypnosis: Therapeutic Approaches to Altered States.* Irvington.

Erickson, M.H., Rossi, E.L., & Rossi, S.I. (1976). *Hypnotic Realities. The Induction of Clinical Hypnosis and Forms of Indirect Suggestion.* Irvington.

Everstine, D.S., & Everstine, L. (1983). *People in Crisis: Strategic Interventions.* Brunner/Mazel

Fisch, R., Weakland, J.H., & Segal, L. (1982). *The Tactics of Change. Doing Therapy Briefly.* Jossey-Bass.

Fisch, R., & Schlanger, K. (1999). *Brief Therapy with Intimidating Cases. Changing the Unchangeable.* Jossey-Bass.

Furman, B., & Ahola, T. (1992). *Solution Talk: Hosting Therapeutic Conversations.* Norton.

Gergen, K.J. (1991). *Therapy as Social Construction.* Sage.

Gershman, N., & Thompson, B.E. (2019). *Prescriptive Memories in Grief and Loss: The Art of Dreamscaping.* Routledge.

Green, D.J. (1995). Persuasive public speaking: How MRI changed the way I preach. In J.H. Weakland & W.A. Ray (Eds.) (1995). *Propagations: Thirty Years of Influence from the Mental Research Institute* (pp. 227–242). Routledge.

Haley, J. (1963). *Strategies of Psychotherapy.* Grune & Stratton.

Haley, J. (1973). *Uncommon Therapy. The Psychiatric Techniques of Milton Erickson, M.D.* Norton.

Haley, J. (1982). The contribution to therapy of Milton H. Erickson, M.D. In J.K. Zeig (Ed.), *Ericksonian Approaches to Hypnosis and Psychotherapy* (pp. 5–25). Brunner/Mazel.

Haley, J. (1985). *Conversations with Milton H. Erickson* (Vols. I–III). Norton.

Hoyt, M.F. (Ed.) (1994). *Constructive Therapies.* Guilford Press.

Hoyt, M.F. (Ed.) (1996). *Constructive Therapies 2.* Guilford Press.

Hoyt, M.F. (Ed.) (1998). *The Handbook of Constructive Therapies.* Jossey-Bass.

Hoyt, M.F. (2000). *Some Stories Are Better Than Others: Doing What Works in Brief Therapy and Managed Care.* Brunner/Mazel.

Hoyt, M.F. (2001). *Interviews with Brief Therapy Experts*. Brunner-Routledge.

Hoyt, M.F. (2009). *Brief Psychotherapies: Principles and Practices*. Zeig, Tucker & Theisen.

Hoyt, M.F. (2017). *Brief Therapy and Beyond: Stories, Language, Love, Hope, and Time*. Routledge.

Hoyt, M.F. (2019a). "No way – you gotta be kidding!": Using ordeals to promote problem stopping. In M.F. Hoyt & M. Bobele (Eds.), *Creative Therapy in Challenging Situations: Unusual Interventions to Help Clients* (pp. 113–120). Routledge.

Hoyt, M.F. (2019b). Going one-down. In M.F. Hoyt & M. Bobele (Eds.), *Creative Therapy in Challenging Situations: Unusual Interventions to Help Clients* (pp. 103–112). Routledge.

Hoyt, M.F., Bobele, M., Slive, A., Young, J., & Talmon, M. (Eds.) (2018). *Single-Session Therapy by Walk-In or Appointment: Administrative, Clinical, and Supervisory Aspects of One-at-a Time Services*. Routledge.

Hoyt, M.F., & Cannistrà, F. (2019) Single-session therapy: A healthful approach to effectively and efficiently solving client problems. *Rivista Sperimentale di Freniatria – The Italian Journal of Mental Health*, 143(1), 73–85.

Hoyt, M.F., & Talmon, M. (Eds.) (2014). *Capturing the Moment: Single Session Therapy and Walk-In Services*. Crown House Publishing.

Hoyt, M.F., Young, J., & Rycroft, P. (Eds.) (2021), *Single Session Thinking and Practice in Global, Cultural, and Familial Contexts: Expanding Applications*. Routledge.

Lankton, S.R., & Lankton, C.H. (1983). *The Answer Within: A Clinical Framework of Ericksonian Hypnotherapy*. Crown House Publishing.

Leonardi, F., & Grassi, G. (2012). *Changing Individual Systems in Order to Obtain Lasting Solutions: Three Brief Strategic Techniques*. Short course presented at Brief Therapy: Lasting Solution Conference sponsored by Milton H. Erickson Foundation, San Francisco, CA.

Leslie, P.J. (2019). *The Art of Creating a Magical Session: Key Elements for Transformative Psychotherapy*. Routledge.

Levy, R.L., & Shelton, J.L. (1990). Tasks in brief therapy. In R.A. Wells & V.J. Giannetti (Eds.), *Handbook of the Brief Psychotherapies* (pp. 145–163). Springer.

Loriedo, C., & Vella, G. (1992). *Paradox and the Family System*. Brunner/Mazel.

Martiny, B.A. (1989). The multidimensional application of therapeutic metaphors in the treatment of depression. In M.D. Yapko (Ed.), *Brief Therapy Approaches to Treating Anxiety and Depression* (pp. 119–150). Routledge.

Nardone, G. (1996). *Brief Strategic Solution-Oriented Therapy of Phobic and Obsessive Disorders*. Jason Aronson.

Nardone, G. (1998). *Psicosoluzioni: Come Risolvere Rapidamente i Più Complicati Problemi della Vita*. BUR.

Nardone, G. (2003). *Cavalcare la Propria Tigre*. Ponte alle Grazie.

Nardone, G., & Balbi, E. (2008). *Solcare il Mare all'Insaputa del Cielo*. Ponte alle Grazie (English translation: *The Logic of Therapeutic Change: Fitting Strategies to Pathologies*. Routledge, 2018).

Nardone, G., & Portelli, C. (2005). *Knowing through Changing: The Evolution of Brief Strategic Therapy*. Crown House Publishing.

Nardone, G., & Portelli, C. (2013). *Ossessioni, Compulsioni, Manie: Capirle e Sconfiggerle in Tempi Brevi*. Ponte alle Grazie.

Nardone, G., & Rampin, M. (2015). *Quando il Sesso Diventa un Problema: Terapia Strategica dei Disturbi Sessuali*. Ponte alle Grazie.

Nardone, G., & Salvini, A. (2018). *The Strategic Dialogue: Rendering the Diagnostic Interview a Real Therapeutic Intervention*. Routledge.

Nardone, G., Verbitz, T., & Milanese, R. (1999). *Le Prigioni del Cibo*. Ponte alle Grazie (English translation: *Prison of Food: Research and Treatment of Eating Disorders*. Karnac, 2005).

Nardone, G., & Watzlawick, P. (1993). *The Art of Change: Strategic Therapy and Hypnotherapy Without Trance*. Jossey-Bass.

Norcross, J.C. (Ed.) (2011). *Psychotherapy Relationships that Work* (2nd ed.). Oxford University Press.

O'Hanlon, W.H. (1987). *Taproots: Underlying Principles of Milton Erickson's Therapy and Hypnosis*. Norton.

O'Hanlon, W.H., & Weiner-Davis, M. (1988). *In Search of Solutions: A New Direction in Psychotherapy*. Norton.

Paoli, B. (2014). *Come Parla un Terapeuta. La Ristrutturazione Strategica*. Franco Angeli.

Pietrabissa, G., Manzoni, G.M., Gibson, P., Boardman, D., Gori, A., & Castelnuovo, G. (2016). Brief strategic therapy for obsessive-compulsive disorder: A clinical and research protocol of a one-group observational study. *BMJ Open*, 6(3): e009118. Doi: 10.1136/bmjopen-2015-009118.

Poerkseng, B. (2001). *Die Gewissheit der Ungewissheit. Gesprache zum Konstruktivismus*. Carl-Auer-Systeme (English translation: *The Certainty of Uncertainty: Dialogues Introducing Constructivism*. Imprint Academic).

Rampin, M. (2004). Counter-delusion stratagems. *Brief Strategic and Systemic Therapy European Review*, 1, 82–87.

Ratner, H., George, E., & Iveson, C. (2012). *Solution Focused Brief Therapy: 100 Key Points and Techniques*. Routledge.

Ruess, N.H. (1997). The nightmare question: Problem talk in solution-focused brief therapy with alcoholics and their families. *Journal of Family Psychotherapy*, 8(4), 71–76.

Rosen, S. (1982). *My Voice Will Go with You. The Teaching Tales of Milton H. Erickson*. Norton.

Schlanger, K., & Krohner, E. (2019). Our clients *are* able and strong: MRI problem-solving brief therapy in action. In M.F. Hoyt & M. Bobele (Eds.), *Creative Therapy in Challenging Situations* (pp. 172–182). Routledge.

Shaw, H.E., & Magnuson, S. (2006). Enhancing play therapy with parent consultation: A behavioral/solution-focused approach. In H.G. Kaduson & C.E. Schaefer (Eds.), *Short-Term Play Therapy for Children* (pp. 216–244). Guilford Press.

Short, D.N. (2021). What is Ericksonian therapy: The use of core competencies to operationally define a nonstandardized approach to psychotherapy. *Clinical Psychology: Science and Practice*, 28(3), 282–292.

Short, D., Erickson, B.A., & Klein, R.E. (2005). *Hope and Resiliency: Understanding the Psychotherapeutic Strategies of Milton H. Erickson, M.D.* Crown House Publishing.

Soo-Hoo, T. (2018). Working within the client's cultural context in single-session therapy. In M.F. Hoyt, M. Bobele, A. Slive, J. Young, & M. Talmon (Eds.), *Single-Session Therapy by Walk-In or Appointment* (pp. 186–201). Routledge.

Soo-Hoo, T. (2019). Beyond reason and insight: The 180-degree turn in therapeutic interventions. In M.F. Hoyt & M. Bobele (Eds.), *Creative Therapy in Challenging Situations* (pp. 193–208). Routledge.

Treccani (2019). *Logica*. www.treccani.it/vocabolario/logica/ (retrieved online 28 February 2019).

von Foerster, H. (1984). On constructing a reality. In P. Watzlawick (Ed.), *The Invented Reality* (pp. 41–62). Norton.

von Glasersfeld, E. (1995). *Radical Constructivism: A Way of Knowing and Learning.* Falmer Press.

Walter, J., & Peller, J. (1992). *Becoming Solution-Focused in Brief Therapy.* Brunner/Mazel.

Watzlawick, P. (1978) *The Language of Change: Elements of Therapeutic Communication.* Norton.

Watzlawick, P. (Ed.) (1984). *The Invented Reality. How Do We Know What We Believe We Know (Contributions to Constructivism)?* Norton.

Watzlawick, P. (1987). If you desire to see, learn how to act. In J.K. Zeig (Ed.), *The Evolution of Psychotherapy* (pp. 91–100). Brunner/Mazel.

Watzlawick, P. (1997). "Insight" may cause blindness. In J.K. Zeig (Ed.), *The Evolution of Psychotherapy: The Third Conference* (pp. 309–317). Routledge.

Watzlawick, P., Beavin, J.B., & Jackson, D.D. (1967). *Pragmatics of Human Communication: A Study of Interactional Patterns, Pathologies and Paradoxes.* Norton.

Watzlawick, P., Weakland, J.W., & Fisch, R. (1974). *Change: Principles of Problem Formation and Problem Resolution.* Norton.

Weakland, J.H., Fisch, R., Watzlawick, P., & Bodin, A.M. (1974). Brief therapy: Focused problem resolution. *Family Process, 13,* 141–168.

Weeks, G.R., & L'Abate, L. (1982). *Paradoxical Psychotherapy: Theory and Practice with Individuals Couples and Families.* Brunner/Mazel.

Yapko, M.D. (1997). *Breaking the Patterns of Depression.* Doubleday.

Yapko, M.D. (2016, December 11). *Keys to Unlocking Depression.* Presentation at Brief Therapy Conference sponsored by Milton H. Erickson Foundation, San Francisco, CA.

Zeig, J.K. (1999). The virtues of our faults: A key concept of Ericksonian therapy. *Sleep and Hypnosis, 1*(2), 129–138.

Zeig, J.K., & Munion, W.M. (1999). *Milton H. Erickson.* Sage Publications.

Chapter 8

Common Errors in Single Session Therapy[1]

"Maybe you don't have a case really, except for the first interview. That would be nice, I think. Every therapist should shoot for one session."
--Jay Haley & Madeleine Richeport-Haley (2003, p. 33)[2]

Single session therapy (SST; Talmon, 1990) is therapy that is approached one-at-a-time (OAAT), with the expectation that there may be only one therapeutic meeting. As Hymmen, Stalker and Cait (2013, p. 61) have written:

SST refers to a conscious approach to make the most of the first session knowing it may be the only session the client decides to attend – not to the situation where there is an expectation that the client[3] will attend multiple sessions but chooses to attend just one.

SST can occur either by appointment or by walk-in. Many clients and clinicians prefer the former route since they can schedule and prepare for the single session (Hoyt et al., 2021, pp. 9–11), whereas others may prefer the walk-in (or, with modern technology, telephone call-in or computer click-in) portal since open-access walk-ins "seize the moment," they work, and they are efficient (Cornish et al., 2020; Bobele & Slive, 2021). Either way, once the client arrives, the SST process is much the same:

1 *Attitude* – treating the session "as if" it might be the only one and hence making the most of every encounter, underpinned by the paramount acceptance that one session could be (and often is!) enough;

2 *Accessibility* – responding in a timely manner without any unnecessary barriers to clients receiving help when they are most ready;

3 *Acting now* – accepting that the best opportunity to address change is NOW, no matter the diagnosis, severity or complexity of the problem; and

DOI: 10.4324/9781003307709-10

4 *Alliance* – asking what clients want to achieve by the end of the session so that the therapist and client can work collaboratively, in the here and now, toward that goal (Hoyt et al., 2021, p. 4).

There is abundant evidence that a single session of therapy is the most common length of treatment and that SST is often effective (Talmon, 1990; Slive & Bobele, 2011; Hoyt & Talmon, 2014; Dryden, 2017; Cannistrà & Piccirilli, 2018/2021; Ewen et al., 2018; Aafjes-van Doorn & Sweeney, 2019; Cannistrà et al., 2020; Hoyt et al., 2018, 2021) with a wide variety of problems (including anxiety, depression, eating disorders, substance misuse, and couple and family conflicts) with clients seen in a wide variety of cultural contexts. There is a clear need and growing support for SST with children and adolescents (e.g., see Duvall et al., 2012; Kachor & Brothwell, 2020; Schleider et al., 2020; Boyhan, 2021; Murphy & Fry, 2021; Bertuzzi et al., 2021) and for the use of a planned single session to augment on-going individual or family work (O'Hanlon & Rottem, 2021). There are also assorted health-psychology single-session programs and protocols (e.g., stress reduction, stop smoking, improve your sleep) with empirical support of efficaciousness.

Various lists of "What are some single session thinking and practice ideas to take with you when you see a client?" have been proposed (see Hoyt et al., 2021, pp. 332–335), all highlighting the importance of having clear treatment goals, evoking client resources, using the therapeutic alliance to encourage clients, planning next steps and keeping an "open door" for possible return visits. Different theoretical approaches have all yielded single-session successes. Careful attention to beginning and ending sessions and to meeting clients in their respective world views, appreciating and working with various cultural nuances, is highly valued.

As Michele Ritterman (2019, p. 163) has written:

> As healers, we will be called upon to do what is necessary at any one moment with any given client. Most important is to understand the client response, more than the therapist intervention. Then we can grasp how the clear representation of the needed image or words, at exactly the right moment and interjected with laser-beam accuracy into the correct spot, sometimes can be as David's stone was destructive to Goliath and as healing as Cupid's arrow to the heart.

To achieve a successful SST, the attitude with which the person approaches the session is a determining factor (Young, 2018, p. 40), since "the therapist's mindset plays a vital role in ensuring that the result can be reached in few sessions – often even one" (Cannistrà, 2021, p. 81). In doing this, focusing on *what works* is usually better, in therapy as in life. However, sometimes it can be helpful to know what to avoid or not to do – and students often ask, "What are the most common errors or mistakes when doing Single Session Therapy?"

How to Reduce the Likelihood that SST Will Be Successful

Inspired by Jay Haley's[4] (1969) ironic[5] "The Art of Being a Failure as a Therapist" and others of his papers, we offer here some ways to avoid successful SST. To aid recognition of counterproductive therapist attitudes and behaviors, we identify them in provocative (and, we hope, humorous) ways. This list is derived from frequently asked questions we have heard when teaching SST workshops. Sometimes clients succeed despite therapists' efforts – but someone with irony deficiency[6] who follows these sardonic strictures will be well on their way to avoiding successful single session (or other brief) therapy.

1 *Tell yourself that you MUST do a one-session SST* – and not that SST is a OAAT "mindset" (see Cannistrà, 2021) and just one possibility. If more time/sessions are needed for a complex or risky case, you can consider it an "SST failure" rather than just that sometimes more than one meeting may be needed – even if the OAAT approach was very helpful in organizing what was accomplished. Keep daunting pressure on yourself. Thoughts like "Damn! I wish Milton Erickson [or Sal Minuchin, or Jay Haley, or...] were here" can be used to keep yourself off balance.

   During SST training workshops many participants worry and ask: "What if I don't help the client in one session? What if the person has several problems to address? Now what?" Our ruthlessly concrete answer: "Do another session." As Jeff Young (2018, p. 40) has written, SST is "an attitude to service delivery," a "sensibility [that] can generate great creative possibilities but that particular misunderstandings risk constraining the widespread potential impact of SST research and thinking." He goes on (2018, pp. 46–50) to discuss four common misunderstandings of SST that you can perpetuate in order to increase the likelihood of failure at every single session:

   1 To see SST as a specific model of therapy rather than as a model of service delivery;
   2 To describe SST as brief therapy rather than as responding to clients' natural help-seeking behavior;
   3 To think that SST is only suitable for clients facing simple problems;
   4 To believe that SST means "only one session."

2 *Along these lines, the therapist can insist on exclusively using his/her favorite model of therapy.* If a client doesn't respond to that particular approach (be it SFBT, narrative therapy, strategic therapy, CBT, EMDR, motivational interviewing, psychodynamics, or whatever) who needs to change? We know that an increasing amount of data confirms that all psychotherapy approaches are more-or-less equivalent in effectiveness (see

Wampold & Imel, 2015) but… "I'm sure mine is still the most effective – and if it doesn't work it must be the client's fault!"

3 *The therapist also can inform a client at the beginning of the session that he/she/they will only have "one shot."* Offering SST apologetically ("I wish I could offer you more sessions, but the Clinic will only authorize one – but maybe one will be enough") can be used to stimulate resistance ("But what if I need more?"), which can then be interpreted to the client as a sign of their bloody-minded lack of motivation.

You can also start with an opening like this:

> Before we begin, I'd like to say something: there are some people who feel that they've got what they needed after one session and want to try to move forward on their own – but there are others who really want help and need more sessions. At the end of today you can tell me if this meeting was enough – or if you think you have a problem that needs real attention.

4 *On the other side, let the client know that you don't expect success in one session. At least, aver that SST is not possible for certain specific problems.* You can mention that some professionals even doubt that SST *is* psychotherapy (see Young & Jebreen, 2020). If a client still indicates that they are ready to change, remind them of the dangers of symptom substitution (despite lack of evidence that symptom substitution really exists – see Tyron, 2008). If a client says that she has sought an SST appointment because she is ready to make some changes, the sophisticated and multi-theoretical therapist can snatch defeat from the jaws of victory and thwart SST success by raising other issues that the client might consider before making any moves: unhappy childhood memories, problems at work, and the uncertainties of the future are usually good candidates. Be sure to check every symptom and to label the person in a specific diagnostic category; requiring further evaluation can successfully avoid ending therapy.

Curb your enthusiasm. As Bregman (2021, p. 259) has written:

> We can't help leaking expectations, through our gazes, our body language and our voices. My expectations about you define my attitude towards you, and the way I behave towards you in turns influences your expectations and therefore your behavior towards me.

A wise man once said, "Whether a person thinks he is going to be a success or a failure, he's probably right." Do your best to reduce positive expectations and hope (see Battino, 2006; Hoyt, 2021).

5 *Disregard reality.* We hasten to caution that to persist with the erroneous belief that difficult problems may not be helped in SST, one will need to be prepared to overlook a large and expanding body of quantitative and qualitative evidence. Fortunately, one need not alter or abandon preconceived notions. In their discussion of how some have dealt with evidence of

single-session successes, O'Hanlon and Wilk (1987, p. ix) helpfully remind us that one could always ask, "It works *in practice* O.K…. but does it work *in theory?*"

Haley (1969, p. 76) was also concerned about reality intruding on theory. He wrote:

> Perhaps the most important rule is to ignore the real world that patients live in and publicize the vital importance of their infancy, inner dynamics, and fantasy life. This will effectively prevent either therapists or patients from attempting to make changes in their families, friends, schools, neighborhoods, or treatment milieus. Naturally they cannot recover if their situation does not change, and so one guarantees failure while being paid to listen to interesting fantasies. Talking about dreams is a good way to pass the time, and so is experimenting with responses to different kinds of pills.

He (Haley, 1969, p. 76) also sagely cautioned: "Avoid the poor because they will insist upon results and cannot be distracted with insightful conversations."

6 *A vague problem and a vague goal also can be used to avoid having the client feel they have achieved their therapeutic aim.* As Hoyt (2000, p. 6) has written, using the metaphor of golf, "It's a long day on the course if you don't know where the hole is." Pam Rycroft (in Hoyt et al., 2021, pp. 325–326) recalls an SST session in which a teenage girl contrasted her weekly visits with a school counselor in which they didn't (as the girl put it) "get to any real stuff" to a productive single session experience she had because "I thought there was no point in bullshittin'!" Beware specificity. Endorse vague, abstract, metaphorical, jargon-laden descriptions of problems. "Self-esteem" is almost always a great place to start.

7 *As a corollary, don't ask the person what they think is a good way to address the problem.* What do they know? Whose therapy is it, anyhow? Asking for the client's theory of change and inquiring about resources and exceptions to the problem can promote client self-empowerment and endanger single-session failure. To be sure of avoiding (at all costs!) the success of an SST we should forget that the "clients' active involvement in the therapeutic process is critical to success" (Bohart & Tallman, 2010, p. 83). Shakespeare clearly wasn't burdened with trying to build a caseload and make a comfortable living when he wrote (in *All's Well that Ends Well*, Act I, Scene 1, line 218), "Our remedies oft in ourselves do lie."

8 *Another way to avoid SST success is, near the end of a session, to look at the clock and say "We still have 10 minutes left. Anything else you want to discuss?"* You won't have time to get into anything new and you'll lose the thrust of the good work that has been done. You can check that nothing essential was missed, and you can use the extra time to talk about

next steps and how they'll use the session, or just compliment the client for being efficient and motivated – but to really avoid SST success, don't stop when you're ahead: start a new topic without enough time.

9 *Avoid small steps.* Behaviorists may talk about "successive approximations to the goal" and Haley (1982, p. 23) wrote: "The small change invariably led to the larger one. As [Milton] Erickson[7] put it, if you want a large change you should ask for a small one." Others interested in rapid change have also advocated encouraging clients to take specific, discrete steps. Goulding and Goulding (1979), for example, would begin a session by asking "What are you willing to change today?" O'Hanlon (1999) advised "Do one thing different." Dryden (2021, pp. 43–45) suggests engaging in a "reflect-digest-act-wait-decide" process in which the client is encouraged to take time to absorb and use what has occurred in a single session before booking another meeting.[8]

But, hey, despite the fact that overreaching usually just leaves us grasping the idea that "Great is the enemy of good," you might hit a "home run" or a "hole in one" (Hoyt, 2000)! So what if the client was really hoping for something much more likely and practical? As Talmon (1990, p. 111) reminds us, "Most of the successful SSTs we have studied do not resemble the demonstrations of master therapists in conferences or books." To increase the chances of failure, jump hard on the first thing you can and attempt dramatic "uncommon therapy" (Haley, 1973) rather than being a pragmatic "constructive minimalist."

10 *Study SST failures.* Talmon (1990, p. 97) also noted, "An important lesson can be learned from each and every failure." In addition to revealing ways to intervene prematurely, careful attention can show us how to leave the client feeling abandoned, how to get the client to reject the therapist, how to overlook when a few more sessions are necessary, and how to avoid feedback. One can fail through ignorance, but it would be even more masterful to realize you've made a mistake… and consciously decide to continue doing it.

11 *Ignore context.* Avoid frameworks and client language that give attention to history, meaning, belief systems, situation, intention, or motivation. To avoid success, rub the client's culture the wrong way. For example, if someone comes from a collectivist background, demand that any solutions entail greater individuation; on the other hand, if their cultural orientation is more individualistic, push intergenerational loyalties (see Soo-Hoo, 2018).

12 *Think that "to resolve a problem" is the only goal of an SST therapist/ therapy.* Clients whose goal is to "get unstuck" and then proceed on their own and who do not expect the therapist to go on the subsequent journey of life with them are to be avoided if the therapist wishes to not spend time needing to locate new clients. "Bait and switch" can be a useful tactic: "You may think that would solve the problem, but we should look deeper"

(see Haley, 1963). The therapist can tell the client that thorough and comprehensive multidimensional diagnosis is necessary before any meaningful discussion of change can take place. If a client claims to have gotten help and wants to leave therapy before you think they should, it's never too late to call them a "dropout," a "borderline," "in denial" or just a "liar." If a client still seems hell-bent on terminating, you can always resort to your trump card: ask him about his mother.

13 *Eschew implementation, supervision, and ongoing training.* Even if some clinicians (and many clients) persist in their interest in SST, failure need not be lost! As Hoyt, Young and Rycroft (2021, p. 339) have advised:

> Single session thinking and practice require both learning and application. Training is the action of teaching and learning a particular attitude, skill or type of behavior. Implementation is the process that turns plans and learning into actions in order to accomplish strategic objectives and goals. If implementation is forgotten, innovative initiatives may appear as "good ideas" but they do not come to fruition.

Don't provide encouragement or administrative support. Keeping trainees away from SST "clinical champions" and case conferences, not aligning SST with the values of organizations and practitioners, and structuring schedules punitively so that doing SSTs results in having to do more and more appointments can help to nip SST before it spreads. Fortunately, Young, Weir and Rycroft (2012), Young, Rycroft and Weir (2014), Renkin et al. (2021), McDonald et al. (2021), Mildred et al., (2021), Fuzzard (2021), and Robinson et al. (2021) have provided a veritable catalogue of successful implementation strategies to be avoided.

Less Could Be More: More Could Be Less

Moshe, if you want to get somewhere fast, go slowly.
--Milton H. Erickson (1978; quoted in Hoyt & Talmon, 2014, p. xix)[9]

For many, the biggest SST error is, paradoxically, to go too fast and to try to cover too much. We have to stay focused. We're not doing a survey. Go slow. Expand accordingly. Sometimes something is "solved" or "resolved" – other times things just get "unstuck" and "processed" and maybe coped with or managed better. One size does not fit all. As Hoyt, Rosenbaum, and Talmon (1992, p. 63) noted:

> The therapist needs to be versatile, innovative, and pragmatic, asking: "What would help this patient today?" Patients may need to begin a process or complete a process; they may need to take hold or to let go; they may need reassurance or confrontation; they may need to look at something

deeply or to shift perspective. [...] Nothing works all the time, but what might work this time?

A lot of longer-term therapies may just be the same series of errors (e.g., no achievable session goal, lack of attention to resources, dubious motivation) repeated over and over. In his "Quiz for Young Therapists," Haley (1977/2010, p. 186) asked "Is it unethical to adopt a theory that change is slow and diffi-cult and every patient must come to therapy several hours a week for many years?" and answered, "Only if the therapist is paid by the hour." In 1990 (pp. 14–15) Haley also opined that "The ideology and practice of therapy was largely determined when therapists chose to sit with a client and be paid for durations of time rather than by results." It is not surprising that in his review of Haley's "The Art of Being a Failure as a Therapist," Len Sperry (2010, p. 79) com-mented: "It is particularly noteworthy that in later years, Haley favored 'rapid recoveries' and 'single-session therapies.'"

SST is not a panacea and is not intended as a replacement for other therapy modalities. It is not an abbreviated form of conventional therapy, nor even a substitute for other "brief" or "time-sensitive" therapies. Other common brief therapy resistances – applicable but not limited to SST – include the belief that "more is better," the myth of the "pure gold" of insight, the confusion of patients' interests with therapists' interests, economic and other pressures, and countertransference and the "need to be needed" (Hoyt, 1985/1995). SST should not be "forced" and is most appropriate for those clients who desire and choose to attend one session (Cummings, 2000).

Conclusion

SST is a common, effective, flexible, increasingly recognized, and important component in the landscape of mental health service delivery. As Hoyt, Young and Rycroft (2021, p. 3) have written:

> The essence of single session thinking is to approach the first session as if it will be the only session, while creating opportunities for further work if it is requested by the client. What emerges is a collaborative, direct, and transparent approach to providing services that puts the client in a very active role in determining the focus and length of the work.

In this article we have endeavored to elucidate some ways therapists may, inad-vertently or intentionally, prevent or undermine the potential effectiveness of SST – including failing to define a session goal, attempting to do too much in one session, ignoring context, and not highlighting clients' abilities and their ideas about what would be helpful. With the expanding interest and need for SST, if therapists avoid these and the other aforementioned errors, includ-ing the mistaken beliefs that one session is intended to completely resolve all problems and that "one-at-a-time" means "only one time," many clients will find a planned single session to be beneficial. It would be an error to offer them that opportunity, would it not?

Notes

1 A version first appeared in *Journal of Systemic Therapies*, 2021, 40(3), 29–41. Used by agreement.

2 © 2002 from *The Art of Strategic Therapy* by Jay Haley. Reproduced by permission of Taylor and Francis Group, LLC, a division of Informa plc.

3 The terms *patient* and *client* are both used throughout the literature (see Hoyt, 2017, pp. 1–5 and pp. 217–218). Physicians and others working in medical settings generally prefer *patient* (emphasizing the medical-model idea of expert-provided diagnosis and treatment), whereas others may favor *client* (to emphasize more collaborative/facilitative/strength-oriented approaches).

4 For those relatively new to the field, Jay Haley (1923–2007) was one of the "first-generation" major developers of family therapy, systemic-strategic therapy, and brief therapy. He was a coauthor of the famous "double-bind" paper (Bateson et al., 1956), the founding editor of the journal *Family Process*, the person who most brought Milton Erickson to wider recognition (e.g., Haley, 1973, 1985) and the author of numerous foundational brief therapy texts. In writing and speech, he was known for his perspicuity, avoidance of obfuscating jargon, and frequent use of satiric-ironic humor. We offer this tongue-in-cheek list as an homage to Haley.

5 *Irony* (*Wikipedia*, retrieved online 24 September 2021) is "a rhetorical device, literary technique, or event in which what on the surface appears to be the case or to be expected differs radically from what is actually the case." The *Oxford English Dictionary* (retrieved 24 September 2021) adds: "A condition of affairs or events of a character opposite to what was, or might naturally be, expected; a contradictory outcome of events as if in mockery of the promise and fitness of things (in French, *ironie du sort*)." According to the *Encyclopedia Britannica*, "The term irony has its roots in the Greek comic character Eiron. [...] The Socratic irony of the Platonic dialogues derives from this comic origin." Aristotle also recommended language that was not obvious and that contained an antithesis that required investigation, "for then there is a learning process or something very like it" (Grube, 1989, p. 89).

6 *Irony deficiency* (*Urban Dictionary*, retrieved online 24 September 2021) is "A common deficiency in which the brain cannot process humor that contains irony." Elsewhere (e.g., Hoyt & Andreas, 2015; Hoyt, 2017, pp. 227–230) we have more generally discussed the use of humor in brief therapy.

7 It is interesting to note that of all Erickson's known cases (see O'Hanlon & Hexum, 1990), one session was the most common length of therapy.

8 Astute readers may note that MRI brief therapists (Fisch et al., 1982) would often counsel "Go slow." The "slow" was intended to co-opt resistance; the operative "go" implied the need to take action. "Reality" may be a socially mediated construction, but as Anderson and Goolishian (1988, p. 377, emphasis added) said: "*We live and take action* in a world that we define through our descriptive language in social intercourse with others." We "perform" (Omer, 1993) or "enact" (Sluzki, 1992) our narratives of the world. Michael White (1989–1990/1992, p. 81) thus wrote: "It is not enough for a person to tell a new story about oneself, or to assert claims about oneself. Instead [...] it is the performance of these texts that is transformative of persons' lives." Sometimes this can be accomplished in one session.

9 Reprinted with kind permission of David Bowman, Crown House Publishing.

References

Aafjes-van Doorn, K., & Sweeney, K. (2019, November 9). The effectiveness of initial therapy contact: A systematic review. *Clinical Psychology Review, 74*, published online. doi: 10.1016/j.cpr.2019.101786

Anderson, H., & Goolishian, H.A. (1988). Human systems as linguistic systems: Preliminary and evolving ideas about the implications for clinical practice. *Family Process, 27*, 371–393.

Bateson, G., Jackson, D.D., Haley, J., & Weakland, J.H. (1956). Toward a theory of schizophrenia. *Behavioral Science, 1*, 251–264.

Battino, R. (2006). *Expectation: The Very Brief Therapy Book*. Crown House Publishing.

Bertuzzi, V., Fratini, G., Tarquinio, C., Cannistrà, F., Granese, V., Giusti, E.M., Castelnuovo, G., & Pietrabissa, G. (2021). Single session therapy for the treatment of anxiety disorders in youth and adults: A systematic review of the literature. *Frontiers in Psychology, 1*(12), 721382. Doi: 10.3389/fpsyg.2021.721382.

Bobele, M., & Slive, A. (2021). An open invitation to walk-in therapy: Opening access to mental healthcare. In M.F. Hoyt, J. Young, & P. Rycroft (Eds.), *Single Session Thinking and Practice in Global, Cultural, and Familial Contexts: Expanding Applications* (pp. 54–65). Routledge.

Bohart, A., & Tallman, K. (2010). Clients: The neglected common factor in psychotherapy. In B.L. Duncan, S.D. Miller, B.E. Wampold, & M.A. Hubble (Eds.), *The Heart and Soul of Change: Delivering What Works in Therapy* (2nd ed., pp. 83–111). American Psychological Association.

Boyhan, P.A. (2021). Complex and challenging issues in SST: Reflections on the past and learnings for the future. In M.F. Hoyt, J. Young, & P. Rycroft (Eds.), *Single Session Thinking and Practice in Global, Cultural, and Familial Contexts: Expanding Applications* (pp. 173–181). Routledge.

Bregman, R. (2021). *Humankind: A Hopeful History*. Little, Brown.

Cannistrà, F. (2021). The vital role of the therapist's mindset. In M.F. Hoyt, J. Young, & P. Rycroft (Eds.), *Single Session Thinking and Practice in Global, Cultural, and Familial Contexts: Expanding Applications* (pp. 77–88). Routledge.

Cannistrà, F., & Piccirilli, F. (Eds.) (2018). *Terapia a Seduta Singola: Principi e Pratiche* (in Italian). Giunti (Published in English as *Single Session Therapy: Principles and Practices*. Giunti, 2021).

Cannistrà, F., Piccirilli, F., D'Alia, P.P., Giannetti, A., Piva, L., Gobbato, F., Guzzardi, R., Ghisoni, A., & Pietrabissa, G. (2020). Examining the incidence and clients' experience of single session therapy in Italy: A feasibility study. *Australian and New Zealand Journal of Family Therapy, 41*(3), 271–282.

Cornish, P.A., Churchill, A., & Hair, H.J. (2020). Open-access single-session therapy in the context of Stepped Care 2.0. *Journal of Systemic Therapies, 39*(3), 21–33.

Cummings, N.A. (2000). The single-session misunderstanding. In *The Collected Papers of Nicholas A. Cummings. Vol. 1: The Value of Psychological Treatment* (J.L. Thomas & J.L. Cummings, Eds.) (p. 77). Zeig, Tucker, & Theisen.

Dryden, W. (2017). *Single-Session Integrated CBT (SSI-CBT)*. Routledge.

Dryden, W. (2021). *Help Yourself with Single-Session Therapy*. Routledge.

Duvall, J., Young, K., & Kays-Burden, A. (2012, November). *No More, No Less: Brief Mental Health Services for Children and Youth*. Policy paper, Ontario Centre of Excellence for Child and Youth Mental Health. Available from www.excellenceforchildrenandyouth.ca.

Ewen, V., Mushquash, A.R., Mushquash, C.J., Bailey, S.K., Haggerty, J.M., & Stones, M.J. (2018). Single-session therapy in outpatient mental health services: Examining the effect on mental health symptoms and functioning. *Social Work in Mental Health*, *16*(5), 573–589.

Fisch, R., Weakland, J.H., & Segal, L. (1982). *The Tactics of Change: Doing Therapy Briefly*. Jossey-Bass.

Fuzzard, S. (2021). Embedding single session family consultation in a national youth mental health service: headspace. In M.F. Hoyt, J. Young, & P. Rycroft (Eds.), *Single Session Thinking and Practice in Global, Cultural, and Familial Contexts: Expanding Applications* (pp. 133–139). Routledge.

Goulding, M.M., & Goulding, R.L. (1979). *Changing Lives through Redecision Therapy*. Brunner/Mazel.

Grube, G.M.A. (1989). *Aristotle on Poetry and Style*. Hackett Publishing.

Haley, J. (1963). The art of psychoanalysis. In *Strategies of Psychotherapy* (pp. 192–201). Grune & Stratton. Reprinted in J. Haley (1969). *The Power Tactics of Jesus Christ and Other Essays* (pp. 11–26). Avon Books; and in M. Richeport-Haley & J. Carlson (Eds.) (2010). *Jay Haley Revisited* (pp. 1–17). Routledge.

Haley, J. (1969). The art of being a failure as a therapist. *American Journal of Orthopsychiatry*, *39*, 691–695. Reprinted in J. Haley (1969). *The Power Tactics of Jesus Christ and Other Essays* (pp. 71–78). Avon Books; and in M. Richeport-Haley & J. Carlson (Eds.) (2010). *Jay Haley Revisited* (pp. 75–91). Routledge.

Haley, J. (1973). *Uncommon Therapy: The Psychiatric Techniques of Milton H. Erickson, M.D.* Norton.

Haley, J. (1977). A quiz for young therapists. *Psychotherapy: Theory, Research and Practice*, *14*(2), 165–168. Reprinted in M. Richeport-Haley & J. Carlson (Eds.) (2010). *Jay Haley Revisited* (pp. 179–187). Routledge.

Haley, J. (1982). The contribution to therapy of Milton H. Erickson, M.D. In J.K. Zeig (Ed.), *Ericksonian Approaches to Hypnosis and Psychotherapy* (pp. 5–25). Brunner/Mazel.

Haley, J. (1985). *Conversations with Milton H. Erickson, M.D.* (Vols. 1–3). Triangle Press.

Haley, J. (1990). Why not long-term therapy? In J.K. Zeig & S.G. Gilligan (Eds.), *Brief Therapy: Myths, Methods, and Metaphors* (pp. 3–17). Brunner/Mazel.

Haley, J., & Richeport-Haley, M. (2003). *The Art of Strategic Therapy*. Routledge.

Hoyt, M.F. (1995). Therapist resistances to short-term dynamic psychotherapy. In *Brief Therapy and Managed Care: Readings for Contemporary Practice* (pp. 219–235). Jossey-Bass [work originally published 1985].

Hoyt, M.F. (2000). A golfer's guide to brief therapy (with footnotes for baseball fans). In *Some Stories are Better than Others* (pp. 5–15). Brunner/Mazel. Reprinted in M.F. Hoyt (2017), *Brief Therapy and Beyond* (pp. 33–43). Routledge.

Hoyt, M.F. (2017). *Brief Therapy and Beyond: Stories, Language, Love, Hope, and Time*. Routledge.

Hoyt, M.F. (2021). The hope and joy of single session thinking and practice. In M.F. Hoyt, J. Young, & P. Rycroft (Eds.), *Single Session Thinking and Practice in Global, Cultural, and Familial Contexts: Expanding Applications* (pp. 29–41). Routledge.

Hoyt, M.F., & Andreas, S. (2015). Humor in brief therapy: A dialogue—Part I. *Journal of Systemic Therapies*, *34*(3), 14–25.

Hoyt, M.F., Bobele, M., Slive, A., Young, J., & Talmon, M. (Eds.) (2018). *Single-Session Therapy by Walk-In or Appointment: Administrative, Clinical, and Supervisory Aspects of One-at-a-Time Services*. Routledge.

Hoyt, M.F., Rosenbaum, R., & Talmon, M. (1992). Planned single-session psychotherapy. In S.H. Budman, M.F. Hoyt, & S. Friedman (Eds.), *The First Session in Brief Therapy* (pp. 59–86). Guilford Press.

Hoyt, M.F., & Talmon, M. (Eds.) (2014). *Capturing the Moment: Single Session Therapy and Walk-In Services*. Crown House Publishing.

Hoyt, M.F., Young, J., & Rycroft, P. (Eds.) (2021). *Single Session Thinking and Practice in Global, Cultural, and Familial Contexts: Expanding Applications*. Routledge.

Hymmen, P., Stalker, C.A., & Cait, C. (2013). The case for single-session therapy: Does the empirical evidence support the increased prevalence of this service delivery model and walk-in services? *Journal of Mental Health, 22*(1), 60–71.

Kachor, M., & Brothwell, J. (2020). Improving youth mental health services access using a single-session therapy approach. *Journal of Systemic Therapies, 39*(3), 46–55.

McDonald, J., Hickey, P., & Wyder, M. (2021). Implementing single session thinking in a public mental health setting in Queensland: Part II – Adapting and integrating single session thinking into an acute care setting. In M.F. Hoyt, J. Young, & P. Rycroft (Eds.), *Single Session Thinking and Practice in Global, Cultural, and Familial Contexts: Expanding Applications* (pp. 110–116). Routledge.

Mildred, H., Hunter, L., Goldsworthy, B., & Brann, P. (2021). Embedding the "Family Oriented Collaboration Utilising Strengths" (FOCUS) clinic in a child and youth mental health service and university partnership. In M.F. Hoyt, J. Young, & P. Rycroft (Eds.), *Single Session Thinking and Practice in Global, Cultural, and Familial Contexts: Expanding Applications* (pp. 278–286). Routledge.

Murphy, M., & Fry, D. (2021). Integrating a single session family therapy approach in two child and youth mental health services. In M.F. Hoyt, J. Young, & P. Rycroft (Eds.), *Single Session Thinking and Practice in Global, Cultural, and Familial Contexts: Expanding Applications* (pp. 287–295). Routledge.

O'Hanlon, B., & Rottem, N. (2021). Single session family consultation (SSFC). In M.F. Hoyt, J. Young, & P. Rycroft (Eds.), *Single Session Thinking and Practice in Global, Cultural, and Familial Contexts: Expanding Applications* (pp. 66–76). Routledge.

O'Hanlon, W.H. (1999). *Do One Thing Different: And Other Uncommonly Sensible Solutions to Life's Persistent Problems*. William Morrow.

O'Hanlon, W.H., & Hexum, A.L. (1990). *An Uncommon Casebook: The Complete Clinical Work of Milton H. Erickson M.D.* Norton.

O'Hanlon, W.H., & Wilk, J. (1987). *Shifting Contexts: The Generation of Effective Psychotherapy*. Guilford Press.

Omer, H. (1993). Quasi-literary elements in psychotherapy. *Psychotherapy, 30*(1), 59–66.

Renkin, C., Alexander, K., & Wyder, M. (2021). Implementing single session thinking in public mental health settings in Queensland: Part I – Introducing single session family consultations into adult inpatient and community care. In M.F. Hoyt, J. Young, & P. Rycroft (Eds.), *Single Session Thinking and Practice in Global, Cultural, and Familial Contexts: Expanding applications* (pp. 101–109). Routledge.

Ritterman, M. (2019). The single stroke: What makes "zingers" zing? In M.F. Hoyt, & M. Bobele (Eds.), *Creative Therapy in Challenging Situations: Unusual Interventions to Help Clients* (pp. 163–171). Routledge.

Robinson, A.M., Harvey, G., McDonald, M., & Honegger, T. (2021). Introducing single session therapy at a university counseling center. In M.F. Hoyt, J. Young, &

P. Rycroft (Eds.), *Single Session Thinking and Practice in Global, Cultural, and Familial Contexts: Expanding Applications* (pp. 143–152). Routledge.

Schleider, J.L., Dobias, M.L., Sung, J.Y., & Mullarkey, M.C. (2020). Future directions in single-session youth mental health interventions. *Journal of Clinical Child & Adolescent Psychology*, 49(2), 264–278.

Slive, A., & Bobele, M. (Eds.) (2011) *When One Hour Is All You Have: Effective Therapy for Walk-In Clients*. Zeig, Tucker, & Theisen.

Sluzki, C.E. (1992). Transformations: A blueprint for narrative changes in therapy. *Family Process, 31*, 217–230.

Soo-Hoo, T. (2018). Working within the client's cultural context in single-session therapy. In M.F. Hoyt, M. Bobele, A. Slive, J. Young, & M. Talmon (Eds.), *Single-Session Therapy by Walk-In or Appointment: Administrative, Clinical, and Supervisory Aspects of One-at-a-Time Services* (pp. 186–201). Routledge.

Sperry, L. (2010). Introduction. In M. Richeport-Haley & J. Carlson (Eds.), *Jay Haley Revisited* (pp. 75–83). Routledge.

Talmon, M. (1990). *Single-Session Therapy: Maximizing the Effect of the First (and Often Only) Therapeutic Encounter*. Jossey-Bass.

Tyron, W. (2008). Whatever happened to symptom substitution? *Clinical Psychology Review, 28*(6), 963–968.

Wampold, B.E., & Imel, Z.E. (2015). *The Great Psychotherapy Debate: The Evidence for What Makes Psychotherapy Work* (2nd ed.). Routledge.

White, M. (1992). Family therapy training and supervision in a world of experience and narrative. In D. Epston & M. White (Eds.), *Experience, Contradiction, Narrative & Imagination: Selected Papers of David Epston & Michael White 1989–1991* (pp. 75–95). Dulwich Centre Publications [work originally published 1989/1990].

Young, J. (2018). Single-session therapy: The misunderstood gift that keeps on giving. In M.F. Hoyt, M. Bobele, A. Slive, J. Young, & M. Talmon (Eds.), *Single-Session Therapy by Walk-In or Appointment: Administrative, Clinical, and Supervisory Aspects of One-at-a-Time Services* (pp. 40–58). Routledge.

Young, J., Rycroft, P., & Weir, S. (2014). Implementing single session therapy: Practical wisdoms from Down Under. In M.F. Hoyt & M. Talmon (Eds.), *Capturing the Moment: Single Session Therapy and Walk-In Services* (pp. 121–140). Crown House Publishing.

Young, J., Weir, S., & Rycroft, P. (2012). Implementing single session therapy. *Australian and New Zealand Journal of Family Therapy, 33*(1), 84–97.

Young, K., & Jebreen, J. (2020). Recognizing single-session therapy as psychotherapy. *Journal of Systemic Therapies, 38*(4), 31–44.

Index

Note: **Bold** page numbers refer to tables, *italic* page numbers refer to figures and page numbers followed by "n" denote endnotes.

accessibility 157
acting now 157
Agency (Efficacy) Questions 31
Alexander, F.: *Psychoanalytic Therapy: Theory and Applications* 82
alliance 4–6, 9, 17, 22, 66, 68n2, 74, 75, 94, 125, 128, 147–148, 158
Analysis Terminable and Interminable (Freud) 16, 53, 81
Anderson, H. 123, 165n8
Andreas, S. 144
anxiety 13, 21, 45, 46, 73, 107, 146, 149, 158
"as if" technique 20–21, 27n40, 46, 128, 145
attempted solution 32, 42, 73, 78, 79, 85, 110, 141, 149
attitude 15, 89, 124, 143, 157, 158, 159, 160, 163
augmentation *vs.* reduction 24n8
aversion 138, 139, 141–144
awareness 10, 78, 93, 111, 129, 138, 140, 143–144, 145, 149

Balbi, E. 138–139; 152n2; *The Logic of Therapeutic Change* 138
Bandler, R. 26n30
Barber, J. 114n14
Bateson, G. 83, *84*, 85, 144, 150
Battino, R. 27n39, 85
Berg, I. K. 30, 84, 105, 137, 143; *The Miracle Method* 117n35
Berra, Yogi 53
The Birth of Venus 109, *109*

Bierce, A. (*The Devil's Dictionary*) 30
Blake, W. 107
Bobele, M. 37, 71, 127
borderline personality disorder 22, 29, 33, 34, 35, 36, 38, 39, 50n38, 107, 163
Bordin, E.S. 23n2
Botticelli 108–109, *109*
Bregman, R. 160
BRIEF (formerly Brief Therapy Practice) 9, 13, 16, 24n11, 59, 101
Brief Family Therapy Center 45, 101, 105, 147
brief therapy 46, 52, 68n2, 84; diagnosis and 28–47; history of 81–113; mindset in 52–67; techniques and logics 70–79; therapeutic relationship 3–23; *see also* logics; single session therapy (SST)
Brief Therapy Conference 32, 62, 83, 86, 92, 99–101
Budman, S.H. 111, 149–150

Cannistrà, F. *109*, *113*, 128, 137, 139, 143; *Single-Session Therapy: Principles and Practices* iii; *Terapia Breve Centrata Sulla Soluzione* iii
case examples 13, 13–14, 16, 19–20, 21–22, 26n30, 27n39, 38–39, 40–41, 45, 45–46, 46, 54, 55, 55–56, 64, 72, 76, 90, 91, 97, 98–99, 107–108, 117, 128–129, 129–130
check-up technique 146

client (term) 4, 5, 8, 10, 23, 25n20, 29, 31, 33, 36, 39, 44, 66, 105, 119n54, 124, 165n3
Clues: Investigating Solutions in Brief Therapy (de Shazer) 136–137
colonization 58, 75
compliments 25n23, 107, 144, 148
constructive therapies 67, 125
context of competence 66–67, 125–126, 126
contract question (Goulding & Goulding) 93–94
Conversations with Milton H. Erickson, M.D. (Haley) 85
couple therapy 130–131
criminal novel 150
Csikszentmihalyi, M. 124
Cummings, N.A. 23n1, 99, 109–110

DBT (Dialectical Behavior Therapy) 39
Dear Doctor technique 148
DeJong, P. 137
depression 29, 35, 37, 40, 45, 107, 142, 143, 147, 158
de Shazer, S. 9, 25n20, 29–31, 33, 37, 40, 45, 47, 79n8, 84, 86, 91, 99–103, 103, 105–106, 112, 125, 135–136, 147, 150; *Clues: Investigating Solutions in Brief Therapy* 136–137; *Keys to Solution in Brief Therapy* 136
diagnosis 4, 28–51, 89, 157, 163, 169
Dilts, R. 62
direct block, of actions 56, 73, 76, 78, 141, 149
dismantling studies 71
distraction 74, 137, 148
Dolan, Y. 99
Dryden, W. 162
DSM (Diagnostic and Statistical Manual) 29–30, 32–34, 47, 49n21, 58
Duncan, B. 6, 143

eating disorder 56, 148, 158
Efran, J. 40
empowerment 58, 126, 129, 130, 161
Endurance (or Coping) Questions 31, 102
Erickson, B.A. 137
Erickson Brief Therapy 15, 32, 63, 78, 110, 146
Erickson, C. 115n20
Erickson, M.H. 9, 14–16, 29, 35, 57, 68n5, 83–85, 84, 123–124, 135,

147–148, 163, 169n7; *Hope and Resiliency* (Short et al.) 85, 137
Erickson-Klein, R. 137
Erikson, E. 108–109
Errors 157–169
Evolution of Psychotherapy Conference 60, 91–92, 95, 99
Exception Questions 13, 26, 29, 31, 44, 144, 161
expectation 52, 58, 67, 129, 157, 160, 165
express and process logic 149–150

fear of help technique 142
Ferenczi, S. 81
Fisch, R. 44, 62, 64, 84, *103*, 127
Flavia (Cheli) 3, 111
von Foerster, H. 140
Frances, A. 29, 48n2
Frank, J. 73, 128
French, T.: *Psychoanalytic Therapy: Theory and Applications* 82
Freud, S. xv, 8, 16, 44, 53–54, 62, 109; *Analysis Terminable and Interminable* 16, 53, 81
Friedman, S. 83, 111

George, E. 13, 24n11, 101
"Getting the Important Work Done Fast" (M.M. Goulding) 94
goal 9, 24n2, 31, 35, 65, 66, 67, 73, 77, 79, 83, 93, 94, 106, *125*, 126, 135, 136, 138, 145, 146, 147, 151, 159, 161, 162, 163, 164
Goethe, J.W. 24n8
Goolishian, H. 71, 169
"Go slow" technique 11, 146, 163, 169n8
Goulding, M.M. 93–94, 98
Goulding, R.L. (Bob) 57, 78, 92, 93–94, 96, 95–98
Grinder, J. 26n30
Gurman, A.S. 111, 150, 159
Gustafson, J. 88–89

Haley, J. 16, 35–36, 49n21, 52, 62, 75, *84*, 111, 135, 157, 159, 161–162, 164, 165n4; *Conversations with Milton H. Erickson, M.D.* xv, 85; *Problem-Solving Therapy* 75; "Quiz for Young Therapists" 164; *Uncommon Therapy* 85, 135
The Handbook of Psychotherapy and Behavior Change 111

Harari, Y.N. 49n17
health maintenance organizations
    (HMOs) 82
Held, B. 32
Hillman, J. 40
Hoffman, L. 38
hope 4, 5, 7, 8, 19, 31, 47, 52, 64, 66,
    72, 73, 77, 117n35, 125, 130, 139,
    148, 160
Hope and Resiliency (Short, Erickson, &
    Klein) 85, 137
how worse technique 142, 144
Hoyt, M.F. 25n23, 100, *109, 113*,
    125–126, 131, 142, 161, 163–164;
    *Brief Therapy and Managed Care:
    Readings for Contemporary Practice* 83;
    Brief Therapy: Principles and Practices
    81; *Interviews with Brief Therapy
    Experts* 100, 111; *The Present is a Gift*
    53; *Some Stories Are Better than Others*
    101
Hubble, M. 38
humor 5, 40, 72, 78, 91, 92, 159,
    165n4, 169n6; *see also* jokes
Hymmen, P. 157
hypochondriacal behavior 141

interval technique 147
irony 169n5; deficiency 159, 165n6
Italian Center for Single Session Therapy
    xiii, xv, 116n26
Iveson, C. 24n11, 25n20, 101

Jackson, D.D. 41, 83
Jennifer (Lillard) 111
jokes 11, 20–21, 53, 57, 61, 64, 71–72,
    90, 101, 104
Jung, C.G. xv

"Keep It Simple, Stupid" ("K.I.S.S.") 45
Kelley, H. 24n8
Keys to Solution in Brief Therapy (de
    Shazer) 136

Lambert, M. 6
Lazarus, A. 6, 74
Leonardi, F. 76
Levy, R.L. 135
Lieberman, J. 30
logbook technique 149
The Logic of Therapeutic Change (Nardone
    and Balbi) 138
logics 69–80, 136, 151; applications
    150–151; aversion 141–143;

awareness 143–144; of belief 138; of
    contradiction 138; direct block 141;
    express and process 149–150; increase
    to reduce 145–146; methods and
    techniques 139–140; of paradox 138;
    relationship, strengthening 147–148;
    resources 144–145; shift the focus
    148–149; similarities and differences
    136–139; small changes (small
    violations) 146–147

managed care 23n1, 83
Martiny, B. A. 142
Matthews, B. 32
measuring the limits technique 144
medical model 4, 28, 29, 36, 40, 65,
    123, 168n3
Meichenbaum, D. 111
memory gallery 150
Mental Research Institute (MRI) xv,
    41–42, 83–86, 110–112
mentor 91–92
Miller, S. 6, 32, 101, 102
mindset 52, 58, 60, 65–67, 67n1, 126,
    129–130, 158–159
Minuchin, S. 57, 83, 115n17
The Miracle Method (Miller & Berg)
    117n35
Miracle Question technique 31, 145

Nardone, G. 19, 20–21, 27n36, 78,
    125, 138–139, 149, 152n2; *The Logic
    of Therapeutic Change* 138
Narrative Therapy 58
National Mental Health Act 82
"9 Logics" 33, 73, 135–151; *see also*
    logics

obsessive doubt 141
obsessive thoughts 129
Occam's Razor 45
OCD 13, 29, 78, 147
O'Hanlon, B. 38, 42, 50n38, 103, 108,
    161–162; *Taproots* 85, 138
one-at-a-time (OAAT) 111, 128, 157,
    159, 165
one-down position 11, 19, 148
one-session therapy 13, 17–18; *see also*
    single session therapy (SST)
operative diagnosis 32
ordeal task technique 71, 137, 142

paradoxical interventions 19, 46, 73, 79,
    129, 138, 145

partitioning 137
Pascal, B. 14
patient (term) 4, 5, 23n1, 30, 34, 36, 47, 68n2, 119n54, 124, 168n3
personality disorders 37–39, 43–44, 50n31, 107
Piccirilli, F. xiii, 92
pivot chord 63–64
planned casual event 145
poor me technique 142
positive psychology 124
post-traumatic stress disorder (PTSD) 41, 82, 107, 118n40
pragmatic approach 38, 76, 127, 162, 163
present (time orientation) 15, 20, 41, 53, 58–59, 66, 83, 93, 108, 123, 145, 157
problem setting 42
Problem-Solving Therapy (Haley) 75
problem talk (*vs.* solution talk) 31, 43, 134n4
Prochaska, J. 18
progression 137
psychoanalysis 81, 127
Psychoanalytic Therapy: Theory and Applications (Alexander & French) 82
psychopathology 54, 56
psychotherapy 6, 12, 18, 28–30, 36–37, 40, 65, 81–83, 110, 124, 127, 135, 145

"Quiz for Young Therapists" (Haley) 164

Rampin, M. 136, 149
Rank, O. 81
Ratner, H. 8, 24n11, 101
readiness, stages of (Prochaska) 18
reality 160–161
reframing 64, 69n23, 71, 142, 145
reorientation 137
resistance 8–10, 15–17, 19, 24n8, 106–107
Ring, K. 24n8
Ritterman, M. 64, 85, 158
ritualistic behavior 141
Rogers, C. 85
Rosenbaum, Robert (Bob) 43, 63, 78, 83, 86, 110, 115n14, 126, 163
Rosen, S. 146
Rossi, E. L. 26n30
Rycroft, P. 161, 163–164

Salvini, A. 125
Satir, V. 71, *84*, 102, 107
scaling questions 31, 145
schizophrenia 29, 34
Schon, D. 42
search for confirmation technique 143
search for exceptions 26, 144, 161
Seligmann, M.E.P. 124
Shelton, J.L. 135
shift the focus 12, 20, 37, 85, 87, 112, 148–149
Short, D. et al.: *Hope and Resiliency* 85, 137
short-term therapy 62, 83, 93, 134; *see also* brief therapy
SIFT 137
single session therapy (SST) 17, 36–37, 126–127, 131; couple therapy case 130–131; errors in 157–165; failures 162; and health 127–128; obsessive thoughts case 129
Single-Session Therapy: Maximizing the Effect of the First (and Often Only) Therapeutic Encounter (Talmon) 126, 128
Skeleton Key Question 31
Slive, A. 127
small changes (small violations) 146–147, 152n4
snap technique 71
solution-building vocabulary 125
solution-focused brief therapy (SFBT) 8, 13, 16, 24n13, 25n23, 26n25, 30–31, 33, 59, 84, 101, 104–105, 113, 139, 143, 144, 148, 159
solution-talk (*vs.* problem-talk) 31, 34, 134n4
Some Stories Are Better than Others (Hoyt) 101
Soo-Hoo, T. 74, 143
South, T. 85
Stalker, C.A. 157
Strupp, H.H. 99, 102
suggestion 137
Sullivan, H.S. 43, 50n40, 64, 83

Talmon, M. 83, 86, 99, 101, 110, 162–163; *Single-Session Therapy: Maximizing the Effect of the First (and Often Only) Therapeutic Encounter* 126, 128
Taproots (O'Hanlon) 85, 138
Tavistock Clinic 134n2

technique 70, 78; *see also specific techniques*
termination 77–78, 93
therapeutic alliance 4, 5, 6, 9, 17, 22,
    23, 66, 67, 68n2, 74, 75, 94, 125,
    126, 128, 147, 148, 158
therapeutic relationship 5, 22, 24n13;
    see also therapeutic alliance
"Therapist Resistances to Short-Term
    Therapy" (Hoyt) 62
time 3, 8, 26n30, 50n40, 53, 58, 59,
    62, 68n2, 69n18, 72, 126, 127,
    131n2, 135, 161–162
Tomm, K. 29–30

Uncommon Therapy (Haley)
    85, 135
utilization 64, 71, 77, 85, 123,
    137, 143

vicious cycle 43

Wampold, B. 33, 71, 123
Watzlawick, P. 8, 33, 59, 64, 76, *84*,
    128, 140, 145
Weakland, J.H. iii, 6, 11, 25n20, 37,
    49n21, 64, 67n1, 83–86, *84*, 91,
    103–105, 146–148
Whitaker, C.A. 45, *87,* 87–92, 110,
    115n17
White, M. 29, 100, 111, 124, 169
Wilk, J. 161
worst fantasy technique 146

Yalom, I. 30
Yapko, M.D. 147
"Yes, but" and "No, but" 10–14, 20,
    27n39, 54
Young, J. 37, 127, 159, 163–164
Young, K. 26n33

Zeig, J. 42, 89, 110, 137

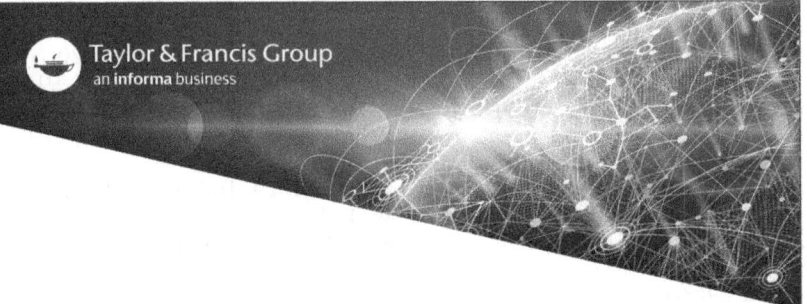
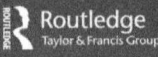
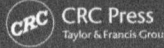